"He Himself bore our sins in His body on the tree, so that we might die to sins and live to righteousness: by His wounds you have been healed."

1 Peter 2:24

YOU NEED TO KNOW...
THE HEALTH MESSAGE

Do you not know that you are God's temple and that God's Spirit dwells in you? If anyone destroys God's temple, God will destroy him, For God's temple is holy and that temple you are.
1 Corinthians 3:16-17

So, whether you eat or drink, or whatever you do, do all to the glory of God. 1 Corinthians 10:31

God Wants You Well!

Beth M. Ley, Ph.D.

BL Publications
Detroit Lakes, MN

BL Publications, Detroit Lakes, MN
For orders call 1-877-BOOKS11
email: blpub@tekstar.com
www.blpbooks.com

Library of Congress Cataloging-in-Publication Data

Ley, Beth M., 1964-
  God wants you well! / Beth M. Ley.
      p. cm.
Includes bibliographical references and index
  ISBN 1-890766-19-4
  1. Healing--Religious aspects--Christianity. 2. Medicine--Religious aspects--Christianity. I. Title.
  BT732 .L46 2001
  234'.131--dc21

                                    2001000334

Printed in the United States of America

All scriptures are taken from The King James Version of the Holy Bible unless otherwise stated.

This book is not intended as medical advice. Its purpose is solely educational. Please consult your healthcare professional for all health problems.

Credits

Cover Design: BL Publications/ Howard Elijah (Signs by Howard, Detroit Lakes, MN)

Cover Art Work: Howard Elijah

Editor: Carter Sandvik

Proofreader: Deborah Brenk

Thank you to all individuals sharing their testimonies for inclusion in this book.

Special thank yous to Melvin and Carol Schultz, Kenneth and Stephanie Scott, Connie Pieske, Margee Boyer, Bryan Ornquist, my mother and the true author of this book, God.

TABLE OF CONTENTS

INTRODUCTION

Nearly one-half of the U.S. population suffers from at least one chronic illness. The estimated cost of health care in the United States for the year 2000 was over $510 billion. By the year 2020, annual medical bills are expected to double to $1.07 trillion. This is an insane amount of money. The average per person cost for an individual with a chronic health problem is over $6,000 a year in doctor visits, prescription medication and hospitalization.

I hate going to the doctor. I hate drugs. The worst thing about spending this money (I think) is that you don't become well. It may help relieve some of your symptoms, but how many people really get well? If you have diabetes, arthritis, elevated cholesterol, asthma, or other chronic health problems, and you are pre-scribed a medication, you (most likely) will have to take it forever...and you will have to continue to pay for it. Medications do not cure you. They don't make you well. They can only help releive some of your symptoms (maybe).

All I have ever wanted was to be well, to be normal–to NOT have to take drugs everyday and make regular trips to the doctor. Since before I can remember, I have been in the "ill half" of the population.

The good news is there is another way. Throughout the Bible God promises us healing. God can and will restore our health. He wants us to be healthy. If we are not feeling well it is difficult to focus on anything else. It is much more difficult to serve Him if we are not well.

And ye shall serve the LORD your God, and He shall bless thy bread, and thy water; and I will take sickness away from the midst of thee. Exodus 23:25

And said, If thou wilt diligently hearken to the voice of the LORD thy God, and wilt do that which is right in His sight, and wilt give ear to His commandments, and keep all His statutes, I will put none of these diseases upon thee, which I have brought upon the Egyptians: for I am the LORD that healeth thee. Exodus 15:26

You see, God wants us to take care of ourselves so we don't get sick in the first place.

I have never been more excited about writing a book (I have written over two dozen books and booklets). Actually, before I began this manuscript, I was starting to feel frustrated with my work. I wondered why my research and writing was not as satisfying as it had been for many years.

I have known for several years that I would write a book for God someday, but felt I wasn't ready. I thought I had so much more research to do on the subject that it would be a long time off in the future before it ever happened. Well, God's timing is certainly not our timing. He showed me how Moses felt he was not ready when God instructed him to go before Pharaoh to ask for the release of the Israelites, and how Jonah probably felt unworthy of his instruction to go to Ninevah to preach of their wickedness.

God's timing is not always our timing.

For several months God really began calling me to write this book. I had not mentally connected my work (writing) and my walk with God. I was praying that He would show me how I could serve Him. His surprising answer was, "I already told you." When the title for this book, *God Wants Us Well*, came to me, I knew that I should get started. When God tells us to do something, it is best not to delay.

In all of the health-related books I have written discussing diet, lifestyle and various nutritional supplements my intent was to help readers improve or restore their health. I know that there is no such thing as a "magic cure" that is going to help everyone. What works wonders for one person may have no effect on someone else with the same health problem. Many people have thanked me for my books telling me how much my research and suggestions helped them, but I knew that there was a missing link.

The missing link is God. We can do nothing without the Father. *I can of mine own self do nothing: as I hear, I judge: and my judgment is just; because I seek not mine own will, but the will of the Father which hath sent me* (John 5:30). We simply cannot do it on our own.

This is a book about faith and obedience.

If we don't take care of ourselves, we will become sick. If we are not obedient, we will suffer the consequences. I have always strongly believed that we have a responsibility to take care of our physical bodies – eat well, eat moderately, and get enough rest and exercise.

I have included the following two scriptures in many of my books:

Do you not know that you are God's temple and that God's Spirit dwells in you? If anyone destroys God's temple, God will destroy him, For God's temple is holy and that temple you are. 1 Corinthians 3:16-17

So, whether you eat or drink, or whatever you do, do all to the glory of God. 1 Corinthians 10:31

My intention for this book is to fill in the missing link: *Therefore, take care to follow the commands, decrees and laws I give you today. If you pay attention to these laws and are careful to follow them, then the Lord your God will keep His covenant of love with you, as He swore to your forefathers... The Lord will keep you free from every disease.* Deuteronomy 7:11-13,15

One of the obstacles I had to deal with before I was willing to start this book, was my own health problems. I asked myself why someone would listen to me and believe what I am telling them about healing when I still have health concerns of my own? I have struggled with asthma since before I can remember. My earliest memories are of being in an oxygen tent in the hospital and in a homemade tent of sorts my mother created with an upside down playpen and a humidifier.

I spent much of my childhood alone as a result of my health problems. I was not allowed to play outside like my two brothers as it seemed I was allergic to the entire outdoors. I was not allowed to visit my friends at their homes in case they had a cat (one of my more severe allergies) or if by chance I would be offered a food I was allergic to. In school I often did not participate in physical education classes because it was too stressful on my lungs. I would just sit on the sidelines and watch. If the class went outside, I just stayed inside by myself. From spring until the first killing frost I really had a hard time. In the winter I was somewhat better, as long as I did not breathe the cold North Dakota air outside.

It is not easy to feel left out (or different or inadequate) especially for a child. Those feeling of rejection can nag you the rest of your life – if you let them.

During my high school years my parents drove me to see a pulmonary specialist in Minneapolis several times, a 10-hour drive from where we lived. He prescribed various medications and inhalers to try to get my asthma under control. I did improve, and was able to participate in cheerleading, and a few other physical activities, but with an inhaler in my hand or close by.

I always had a hard time with the idea that I had to take a drug every 12 hours in order to breathe. I never went anywhere without my inhaler. I had them all over the house – the kitchen, the bedroom, the bathroom, the office, the car, at least two different coat pockets, and of course, my handbag or briefcase.

In college, my health deteriorated. My grass allergy got so severe that I had hives from head to toe during summer school one year. I could not walk in grass with shorts on even if I was wearing shoes and socks. The hives itched horribly and it was not a pretty sight. I was so desperate (as much as I hated doctors and hospitals) that I went to the emergency room begging for relief. The staff said there was nothing they could do and that

I would just have to figure out what I was allergic to and avoid those things. I knew exactly what I was allergic to... the outdoors.

That summer vacationing at the lake, my brothers took turns carrying me from the cabin to the dock. That was about the last straw for me. I started researching and reading everything I could concerning hives, allergies and asthma. I changed my diet. I was already a vegetarian, but didn't really know what I was doing. I was just not eating meat. I started taking alfalfa as a cleanser and detoxifier, MaHuang as a natural bronchial dilator, B Complex Vitamins, Vitamin C, essential fatty acids and whatever else I thought might help. I achieved some success, but not to the extent that I could stop taking my medication without my lungs becoming constricted. In the process, I became fascinated with the whole idea of nutritional supplements and approaching health from a "natural" position. I ended up changing my degree program from physical therapy to scientific and technical writing because I knew without a doubt that I wanted to write about health.

After college I was blessed with the ability to work for various companies involved in the natural health and nutritional supplement industry, where I was able to continue my quest for health. I could do what I enjoyed the most – research and write about health. In all my years of researching the newest nutritional supplements and trying just about everything, I never felt like I really helped my lung situation as I was never able to discontinue taking drugs. I hated taking them, but without the ability to inhale oxygen without effort,

I felt I had no choice.

Over the years my concerns about the drug side effects, toxicity, long term effects on my liver, risks for pregnancy, etc., have increased. I know I have helped a great number of people with their health problems through my books, but feeling like a failure in my own search for wellness, I couldn't help but ask God why He would want me to write a book about healing.

It is not easy to do all that God asks of us. We often analyze the situation and think, "I can't do that." It is true, we cannot – without God. It is difficult to change. It is our human nature to resist change. It is our nature to dislike anything that takes us out of our comfort zone.

The Apostle Paul wrote: *And lest I should be exalted above measure through the abundance of the revelations, there was given to me a thorn in the flesh, the messenger of Satan to buffet me, lest I should be exalted above measure. For this thing I asked the Lord three times, that it might depart from me. And he said unto me, My grace is sufficient for thee: for my strength is made perfect in weakness. Most gladly therefore will I rather glory in my infirmities, that the power of Christ may rest upon me. Therefore I take pleasure in infirmities, in reproaches, in necessities, in persecutions, in distresses for Christ's sake: for when I am weak, then am I strong.* 2 Corinthians 12:7-10

Sometimes God does not remove our thorns for reasons that we cannot yet fully understand. He wants us to remember the good things he has done for us, trials he has brought us through, and lessons we have learned. Often, He is just teaching us that we are to lean on Him, and trust *Him, instead of our own abilities*. When God reminds us that we can do nothing without Him, it can be very humbling. Paul wanted a "quick fix" for his thorn, and God told him that His grace was sufficient.

We need to learn to put all our trust in God. He always has a purpose, even though we may not understand the things He is trying to show us at the time.

The definition of faith is trusting in God, *in spite* of our circumstances. If our circumstances were without trials, what would we need faith in God for? We must be very careful not to think that we don't need God, because that is when He just may show us how much we do!

Through our experiences and suffering, we learn to be more compassionate to others. For example, if we have experienced chronic pain in our life, we are much more compassionate to others who are in chronic pain. Only if we have experienced the misery of cancer, can we truly know the difficulty and pain of one who has cancer.

God comforts us in our tribulations. In the world we will all suffer much in our physical weakness, but through His son, Christ Jesus, we can have complete peace. Christ sympathizes with us and suffers with us. He experienced all the sin and suffering of the entire world as he died on the cross. He knows exactly what we are going through because He is experiencing it with us. When we hurt, He hurts.

God wants us to comfort others in need by communicating our own experiences with His divine goodness and mercy. When God blesses us, it is intended not only to bring us joy, but also to be used to help others.

Throughout the book I have included testimonies and stories sent to me from special friends and from individuals that I have never met who were somehow inspired to write to me. I hope that they help you see how God is truly working in the lives of others.

Blessed be God, even the Father of our Lord Jesus Christ, the Father of mercies, and the God of all comfort; Who comforteth us in all our tribulation, that we may be able to comfort them which are in any trouble, by the comfort wherewith we ourselves are comforted of God. For as the sufferings of Christ abound in us, so our consolation also aboundeth by Christ. And whether we be afflicted, it is for your consolation and salvation, which is effectual in the enduring of the same sufferings which we also suffer: or whether we be comforted, it is for your consolation and salvation. And our hope of you is stedfast, knowing, that as ye are partakers of the sufferings, so shall ye be also of the consolation. 2 Corinthians 1:3-7

Beloved, I wish above all things that thou mayest prosper and be in health, even as thy soul prospereth. 3 John 1:2

God Wants You Well!

God Loves Us

God created us for two purposes. First to love us and have fellowship with us, second so that we could serve him. *Knowing that of the Lord, ye shall receive the reward of the inheritance: for ye serve the Lord Christ.* Colossians 3:24

God will do whatever it takes to draw us to him. He wants a personal relationship with us. He wants us to spend time with Him, talk to Him, listen to Him and depend on Him for everything.

God can use sickness and disease in many ways. It is important to understand that while we may not always understand why we have health problems, He does not want us to be ill for the sake of our suffering.

Sometimes God will use healing to get your attention and show you His love and His character. When Christ was on earth, His healing power was also an affirmation of His ability to forgive sins.

But that ye may know that the Son of man hath power upon earth to forgive sins, (he said unto the sick of the palsy,) I say unto thee, Arise, and take up thy couch, and go into thine house. Luke 5:24

Daryl had been passing blood in his urine for about a month and intended to go to the doctor but just kept putting it off. He attended an evangelistic meeting one night and the pastor there prayed for him. He felt enveloped in a cloud of love and since then has not had blood in his urine. This caused Daryl to really take God seriously in his life and his desire to know Him better became paramount. He realized the love God has for all people, which He showed to him personally, and he wanted more. He continued in his walk and now is a pastor doing God's work.

Christy was only three years old when she fell into a basement landing on the hard concrete. She was unable to walk. Since it was very late, her distressed parents took her home and put her to bed. Early the next morning her parents found that she was unable to move her legs and she was in great pain. Her mother, Cindy, went to the telephone to call the clinic. They had prayed for her that night asking God to heal their little girl and they prayed again several times in the morning. Their six-year-old son, Michael, was sitting right beside Christy. His father said to Michael, "Why don't you lay hands on your sister and pray for her to be healed." So he did. Immediately, Christy bolted up from the couch and ran all over the house. She was instantly and completely healed and never had a problem thereafter. This really made the entire family take note of God's divine love, and showed them *that He is not a respecter of persons. He can hear and work through a child's sincere prayer as well as through an eloquent one delivered by a seasoned prayer warrior. God hears our prayers and none are more important than any other to God. This, of course, did not affect the child as much as it did the parents, whose lives were changed. They continued in their walk with God and now both of them pray regularly for others to be healed and have seen much fruit in their ministry. Christy now attends Oral Roberts University and plays on the volleyball team. Her brother, Michael, attends the same school.*

God May Use Illness to Get Our Attention

As Christians, when we are not walking in God's will, He will let us know. When we have our backs turned on God (rebellion), and are "doing our own thing," we may wonder where God is. But Hebrews 13:5 tells us that God said, *I will never leave thee, nor forsake thee.* This promise was made to Joshua (1:5) when he was in a difficult situation, but belongs to all of God's children. It contains the sum and substance of all the promises. *I will never, no, never leave thee, nor ever forsake thee.*

If we are ignoring God, however, He may need to get our attention. He probably has hundreds of ways of doing this – little things like a close call or two while driving, or at work, sending people into your life, the Holy Spirit prompting you not to go certain places you maybe don't belong, or encouraging you to stop a rebellious behavior, etc. But if these fail, and we continue to ignore Him and fall into disobedience, He may get our attention with the suffering we experience through a health problem, accident or other trial. God does not necessarily cause these these things to happen, but He may allow them, if they meet His purpose.

He may be telling us to slow down (or maybe to wake up) and pay attention to Him. He may be telling us to change our focus and put it onto Him instead of ourselves.

The bottom line is God is a jealous God.

For thou shalt worship no other god: for the LORD, whose name is Jealous, is a jealous God. Exodus 34:14

If God is not first in our lives, He may allow our sin to come to fruition. He may allow circumstances to happen that will make us so miserable that we can do nothing but cry out to Him. God is always there waiting to rescue us. In the midst of "the trial," this may seem cruel, but in most cases if we look back on our lives and recognize the times when this may have happened, we will see what God was trying to do and it will make more sense.

I certainly think He got Paul's (then, still called Saul) attention when he blinded him for three days (Acts 9:9). Prior to this, Saul had been running around *breathing murderous threats against the Lord's disci-*

ples. He was putting men and women in prison because they were Christians or *belonging to the Way* as they called it then (Acts 9:1-2). I would guess that God was getting a little upset with this guy! You do not want God to be angry with you. Why does He get angry? Because of sin and disobedience.

Remember, Satan is looking to destroy us. This, combined with the poor choices we may make when we are not in obedience, can result in a car accident, loss of a job, cancer, a broken leg, even migraine headaches or some type of chronic disease. God will use this to reveal Himself to us as our source of hope and help. God has to be first in our lives.

We need to acknowledge that we are sinners and repent of those sins before we can be forgiven and expect to be healed:

> *But their scribes and Pharisees murmured against his disciples, saying, 'Why do ye eat and drink with publicans and sinners?' And Jesus answering said unto them, 'hey that are whole need not a physician; but they that are sick. I came not to call the righteous, but sinners to repentance.'* Luke 5:30-32

God may also use healing to bring someone into repentance. Healing is an awesome gift from God which can humble us and show us of the magnitude of His love, and the importance of our obedience to Him.

God May Allow Illness as a Punishment for Sin

"Self-help" books are extremely popular today. From a Christian standpoint, this is an oxymoron. The bottom line is that we cannot help ourselves. Only God can help us. One of the things I have seen stressed in self-help books is that Illness and health problems *are not a result of sin.*

One author wrote: *Another of our misconceptions about disease is that it is a punishment for our sins. Generally, this guilt has no basis in reality but has been instilled in us by parents, teachers and other authority figures in our lives...* (Siegel) Reading this, I could only think, "Oh, really? This seems contrary to scripture."

Of course, NOT ALL sickness and disease is a result of sin, however, there are dozens of examples in the Bible showing us that God does allow sickness as punishment for sin. We all have sinned. If you think you have no sin in your life, humbly pray and ask God to reveal it to you. He will.

If we say that we have no sin, we deceive ourselves, and the truth is not in us. 1 John 1:8

There is no soundness in my flesh because of thine anger; neither is there any rest in my bones because of my sin. For mine iniquities are gone over mine head: as an heavy burden they are too heavy for me. My wounds stink and are corrupt because of my foolishness. I am troubled; I am bowed down greatly; I go mourning all the day long. For my loins

15

are filled with a loathsome disease: and there is no soundness in my flesh. Psalm 38:3-7

The LORD will strengthen him upon the bed of languishing: thou wilt make all his bed in his sickness. I said, LORD, be merciful unto me: heal my soul; for I have sinned against thee. Psalm 41:3-4

There is no question that we reap what we sow. *Even as I have seen, they that plow iniquity, and sow wickedness, reap the same* (Job 4:8). Our God is a holy God and cannot tolerate sin. If we know we have sin in our life, and continue to go on sinning, it is against the character of God to bless us. Good health is a blessing.

All thy lovers have forgotten thee; they seek thee not: for I have wounded thee with the wound of an enemy, with the chastisement of a cruel one, for the greatness of thine iniquity, because thy sins were increased. Why criest thou for thy hurt? thy pain is incurable: for the greatness of thine iniquity, because thy sins were increased, I have done these things unto thee. Jeremiah 30:14-15

The Divine principal "we reap what we sow" is still truth. However, with the New Covenant (John 1:12-17), things are not exactly as they were in the Old Testament. Today, we bring punishment upon ourselves as Satan tempts us and we choose to fall.

If we are not obedient, we will suffer the consequences. In addition to illness, God may allow many other consequences to occur in our lives because of sin or disobedience so that we may learn from our mistakes. Look what happened to certain Kings who did not rule according to His will:

Jehoram, King of Judah

God was displeased with the evil brought into Jerusalem by Jehoram, who reigned for eight years in Jerusalem, *because he had forsaken the LORD God of his fathers.*

And there came a writing to him (King Jehoram) from Elijah the prophet, saying, 'Thus saith the LORD God of David thy father, Because thou hast not walked in the ways of Jehoshaphat thy father, nor in the ways of Asa king of Judah, But hast walked in the way of the kings of Israel, and hast made Judah and the inhabitants of Jerusalem to go a whoring, like to the whoredoms of the house of Ahab, and also hast slain thy brethren of thy father's house, which were better than thyself: Behold, with a great plague will the LORD smite thy people, and thy children, and thy wives, and all thy goods: And thou shalt have great sickness by disease of thy bowels, until thy bowels fall out by reason of the sickness day by day.'

Moreover, the LORD stirred up against Jehoram the spirit of the Philistines, and of the Arabians, that were near the Ethiopians: And they came up into Judah, and brake into it, and carried away all the substance that was found in the king's house, and his son's also, and his wives; so that there was never a son left him, save Jehoahaz, the youngest of his sons. *And after all this, the LORD smote him in his bowels with an incurable disease. And it came to pass, that in process of time, after the end of two years, his bowels fell out by reason of his sickness: so he died of sore diseases.* 2 Chronicles 21:12-19

Uzziah, King of Judah

King Uzziah stepped outside of his kingly duties by going inside the temple to burn incense which was the consecrated responsibility of the priests.

*But when he (King Uzziah – also called Azariah in 2 Kings 14: 21 and 15:4) was strong, his heart was lifted up to his destruction: for he transgressed against the LORD his God, and went into the temple of the LORD to burn incense upon the altar of incense. And Azariah the priest went in after him, and with him fourscore priests of the LORD, that were valiant men: And they withstood Uzziah the king, and said unto him, It appertaineth not unto thee, Uzziah, to burn incense unto the LORD, but to the priests the sons of Aaron, **that are consecrated to burn incense**: go out of the sanctuary; for thou hast trespassed; neither shall it be for thine honour from the LORD God. Then Uzziah was wroth, and had a censer in his hand to burn incense: and while he was wroth with the priests, the leprosy even rose up in his forehead before the priests in the house of the LORD, from beside the incense altar. And Azariah the chief priest, and all the priests, looked upon him, and, behold, he was leprous in his forehead, and they thrust him out from thence; yea,*

himself hasted also to go out, because the LORD had smitten him. And Uzziah the king was a leper unto the day of his death, and dwelt in a several house, being a leper; for he was cut off from the house of the LORD: and Jotham his son was over the king's house, judging the people of the land. Now the rest of the acts of Uzziah, first and last, did Isaiah the prophet, the son of Amoz, write. So Uzziah slept with his fathers, and they buried him with his fathers in the field of the burial which belonged to the kings; for they said, He is a leper: and Jotham his son reigned in his stead.
2 Chronicles 26:16-23

Today, we have kingly and priestly duties as well. We are not to go outside of what God has called us to do. God intends for us to serve Him in the way that He has called us. Some people (such as kings) have the financial resources to get the work (carried out by the workers or priests) done. If God is calling you to tithe, you should be obedient and not try to be a worker instead.

Leviticus 27:32 (*And concerning the tithe of the herd, or of the flock, even of whatsoever passeth under the rod, the tenth shall be holy unto the LORD*) and Dueteronomy 14: 22-29 tell us how to tithe – to give back to the Lord what is already His. If we do not tithe or do not tithe correctly, something is likely to happen. The car or the washing machine may break down causing you to spend the money on repairs or illness may create not only costly doctor and hospital bills, but suffering as well. If we don't obey, by tithing, He has the power to create circumstances which can take money away from us.

King Herod

King Herod refused to give glory to God for providing for the people. Dressed in the royal apparel of a dazzling silver bright robe, Herod sat upon his throne and delivered a public address to his subjects. When the people acclaimed him as a god, he did not deny it. Immediately, Herod was struck with violent pains, was carried out and died five days later. (NIV notes on Acts 12: 21–Josephus, Antiquities, 19.8.2)

And immediately the angel of the Lord smote him, because he gave not God the glory: and he was eaten of worms, and gave up the ghost. Acts 12:23

Note that God used the Kings as examples to the people. Punishment does not just happen to kings. We are all alike in God's eyes and just as responsible as they were to obey him.

Fools, because of their transgression, and because of their iniquities, are afflicted. Their soul abhorreth all manner of meat; and they draw near unto the gates of death. Then they cry unto the LORD in their trouble, and he saveth them out of their distresses. He sent his word, and healed them, and delivered them from their destructions. Oh that men would praise the LORD for his goodness, and for his wonderful works to the children of men! Psalm 107:17-21

It is good for me that I have been afflicted; that I might learn thy statutes. Psalm 119:71

The Good News!

Our God is a forgiving God, and after a time of discipline, if we repent from our sin, God often promises to restore our health.

If my people, which are called by my name, shall humble themselves, and pray, and seek my face, and turn from their wicked ways; then will I hear from heaven, and will forgive their sin, and will heal their land. 2 Chronicles 7:14

For the iniquity of his covetousness was I wroth, and smote him: I hid me, and was wroth, and he went on frowardly in the way of his heart. I have seen his ways, and will heal him: I will lead him also, and restore comforts unto him and to his mourners. Isaiah 57:18

O LORD my God, I cried unto thee, and thou hast healed me. Psalm 30:2

God wants us to seek Him for our redemption.

Call unto me, and I will answer thee, and will show thee great things, and difficult, which thou knowest not. For thus saith Jehovah, the God of Israel, concerning the houses of this city, and concerning the houses of the kings of Judah, which are broken down to make a defense against the mounds and against the sword; while men come to fight with the Chaldeans, and to fill them with the dead bodies of men, whom I have slain in mine anger and in my wrath, and for all whose wickedness I have hid my face from this city: Behold, I will bring it health and cure, and I will cure them; and I will reveal unto them abundance of peace and truth. Jeremiah 33:3-6

This discipline is in love:

My son, despise not the chastening of the LORD; neither be weary of his correction: For whom the LORD loveth he correcteth; even as a father the son in whom he delighteth. Proverbs 3:11-12

As many as I love, I rebuke and chasten: be zealous therefore, and repent. Revelation 3:19

My son, regard not lightly the chastening of the Lord, Nor faint when thou art reproved of him; For whom the Lord loveth he chasteneth, And scourgeth every son whom he receiveth. It is for chastening that ye endure; God dealeth with you as with sons; for what son is there whom his father chasteneth not? Hebrews 12:5-7

The following is a story about my friend, Jeannie. I have known her for almost 12 years so I know her story personally. I witnessed much of what she went through. I always told her that God must have something really important planned for her in order to keep her alive. The fact that she is still alive is a miracle in itself.

Jeannie wrote:

God has always given me everything I ever asked for. He let me make all my own mistakes so that I could learn from them. He has rescued me over and over again. I have kept Him so busy it's hard to believe that He had time to deal with anyone else. I can see how much He loves me. All I have learned and the wisdom I have gained, is just amazing. I know God wants me to share what I have learned with others. If I didn't, it would all be a waste.

I have never had wealth of my own, but for some reason God allowed me to live the life of the rich and famous and to be able to mingle among history makers and movers and shakers. This taught me a lot about human nature and temptation.

I grew up in northern California a skinny, ugly kid. Right after graduating from high school, I was in a motorcycle accident which left me with a crushed left side including my leg, arm and face. My entire body needed pins first, then plastic surgery – particularly my nose where the bridge had collapsed. I had dozens of surgeries within a few years. The day after I got the cast off my leg, I moved to New York and somehow got a job as a Playboy Bunny.

About 10 years later, while I was living on a yacht and sailing around the world, I heard about a new grafting procedure for cosmetic surgery which someone had recommended to me upon seeing my nose. I contacted a friend of mine in the U.S. who was a photographer at Playboy and asked him if he knew a good plastic surgeon who could graft my nose. He referred me to one of the world's most famous plastic surgeons. Around that time, if anyone in Hollywood had any work done, he was the one doing it. Upon returning to this country I went to see him, got my nose grafted from my ears and got silicone breast implants not long after. Soon, I was having a relationship with my doctor. I began working for him in his medical building in Los Angeles and socialized with just about every well-known celebrity in the industry at that time. Most weekends were spent at the Playboy Mansion. I was surrounded by beauty, money, power and fame and was given the e-ticket ride through Tinseltown.

Since I coordinated the operating room schedule in my boyfriend's office, I was always in contact with women who wanted breast enhancement. I believed at the time that breast implants were safe, and I assured hundreds of women they had nothing to worry about. Everyone in Hollywood was getting them – I had them, too. It was also true that physical beauty in this world got you anywhere – and I went everywhere with anybody who was anyone.

In 1988, I had a problem with my implants rupturing, so the new highly experimental polyurethane foam-covered implants filled with silicone, replaced the leaking implants. These became highly popular with all the Playboy models because of their natural

24

looking appeal and the lower rate of contracture of the capsule.

By 1991, I developed a rheumatoid condition which got so bad that I couldn't carry anything. Straightening out my right arm was impossible, and I was having trouble walking. I had trouble bathing myself, dressing myself and combing my hair which is very long – between my bottom and my knees. From 1992 to 1994 I was chronically sick with colds, flu, strep throat, fainting spells, vomiting and I still had no use of my right arm. I had 14 inches cut off of my tangled hair because I could no longer care for it. I was photosensitive and had ulcers all over. I was diagnosed with lupus and had various other health problems as well – pericarditis, and a cervical ablation (class 5 – meaning a pre-cancerous condition that required surgery).

In 1994, a friend of mine was questioning the safety of the implants and was concerned about some symptoms I was having and asked me to ask my now ex-boyfriend, the plastic surgeon, if there might be a problem. I assured him they were perfectly safe. Five minutes after this, I picked up a book and opened to a page that read something like, "Do not put a foreign object into your body. This defies God's law. The body will reject it and is likely to develop an autoimmune illness such as lupus." It was like God whacked me on the side of the head.

I found out women were dying from these implants. A woman I knew had asked me about the safety of the implants telling me her's had ruptured and that she was very sick. She thought her health problems were due to the implants, but I reassured her of their safety. When I tried to contact her just a few months later, she had died – at age 42 leaving behind two children and her husband. After I discovered the cause of my illness, I promised her husband that I would inform all women who were considering implants about the risks, and I profusely apologized for my ignorance and lack of compassion.

I was referred to a news reporter by a friend of mine who convinced me I needed to get the implants out as soon as possible. Ater my conversation with her, I had a mammogram. The report indicated intact implants. The truth is: there were none. My body ate them! COMPLETELY! The polyurethane covering was GONE; the silicone sack the silicone gel was contained in, was gone as well. In June 1994, the moment the surgeon's hand pierced my skin with a knife, loose silicone ran down the operating room table onto the floor! It took over 10 hours to attempt to sponge as much silicone out of my body as they could. Saline implants were reinserted as my silicone level was so toxic that it didn't matter, and my natural body was an unnatural wreck after three previous disastrous breast surgeries.

My health improved overnight, but symptoms remain and probably will for a lifetime. As far as the emotional pain involved, I don't even want to go there, but I can honestly say the feeling of betrayal and abandonment was unmeasured to any experience in comparison in my lifetime. The cost initially to get breast implants: $5000. The cost this time with a complication: $15,000. Future costs: ???$$$. Emotional cost: Priceless. No amount of money could fix me now. Health insurance doesn't cover it either.

For my business, I had secured a number of toll free vanity numbers. One of them was 800-BEAU-TY3. Some time previous to my owning the number, a plastic surgeon had advertised a "safe breast augmentation procedure" and to call 800-BEAUTY3 for more information. Well, that number rings to my office. Anyone who calls looking for more information about safe breast augmentation, gets the truth! I have probably talked 500 women out of getting this surgery. I just thank God that He is using me in this way.

In 1996 I developed uterine fibroid tumors (the size of two grapefruits) that nearly killed me. They were discovered when I began to hemorrhage out of control. I steadfastly refused to have a hysterectomy as I was advised to do by more than one doctor. I instead prayed for a miracle. In just a few days, the author of this book had seen a news report about an experimental surgery called embolization of fibroids at UCLA that "had my name on it." She called me to inform me of it and I became the first woman in the United States to have this procedure performed. It was a 100% successful, miraculous recovery!! Praise God! Because of my success with the procedure, the 600,000 women every year with fibroids can have the same done and avoid a hysterectomy as well.

The reason that I know it is so important for us to follow God's will is that we don't ultimately understand what our path will be. God has the 20/20 hindsight that we as humans don't possess. It seems that my sight seems to be from my hind all right. No wonder I can't see at all! It seems that all of the "opportunities" that have befallen me, namely, the terrible motorcycle accident, the breast implant saga, tumors, and numerous other health and personal problems, all turned out to be positive, wonderful things because my own problems were solved. I grew, and helped others to do the same. Someone was always there for me. It's like a torch of light that you pass onto the next person and they give the gift next. God chose my destiny because he knew I would solve the "problem" which in turn, helped someone else. I accept my responsibility seriously. If you learn something wonderful, why keep it to yourself? Are we not here to serve humanity, to make this world a better place? We have much work to do here, and I believe with all my heart that I am still here because I accept that responsibility, embrace it, and consider it a privilege to do God's work.

Recently, I found out I no longer have use of my left internal jugular vein, probably due to a birth defect. A noisy venous hum brought this to my attention in 1998 which prompted further testing. Miracles do happen to me, and if I am to overcome this obstacle as well, then I'm sure the answer for me will not be just for me alone. To discover solutions and impart them to others is a gift to the giver and the receiver alike. Rediscovery solidifies the learning experience.

I have learned to stay in the moment more as I cannot change the past other than to ask for forgiveness, and I cannot predict the future, because only God knows that. The connection to God exists in the moment. That's why we need to be in constant communication with God. If our life is in Him, His life is in us.

God has always given me exactly what I prayed for. I'm always wanting something and getting what I want. I would be very specific and God would grant me my wishes – just enough to hang myself with! Now I know that I should have asked Him for HIS WILL. I know it's His way or no way. Through my experiences I do believe I have moved up the spiritual food chain. I have learned that by looking for a higher meaning, shades of perspective change that prepare us for lessons beyond our lifetime. If we take care of our bodies we last longer. If we take care of our souls we live forever.

God does have specific guidelines that are for our own good. In Leviticus 19:28, He says: Ye shall not make any cuttings in your flesh for the dead, nor print any marks (NIV says tattoos) upon you: I am the LORD.

With many of these Old Testament guidelines it is difficult to know what falls under the law and what does not. The bottom line is that if the Holy Spirit convicts you that something is not right to do, you had better listen.

Leviticus 19:28 could also apply to things like piercing your ears or other body parts and dying your hair. There are also passages in the New Testament that relate to this: *That women adorn themselves in modest apparel, with shamefacedness and sobriety; not with braided hair, or gold, or pearls, or costly array* (1 Timothy 2:9). *Whose adorning let it not be that outward adorning of plaiting the hair, and of wearing of gold, or of putting on of apparel* (1 Peter 3:3).

When considering these things ask yourself if it brings glory to God or to yourself? These scriptures do not say we are not to wear gold or pearls, they stress that our beauty should come from within and that we should show modesty.

Be very careful not to convict others who may do these things. If you do, you are condemning them under the law, which is very dangerous. Remember that God works differently in each of us – in different timing.

Judge not, that ye be not judged. For with what judgment ye judge, ye shall be judged: and with what measure ye mete, it shall be measured to you again. And why beholdest thou the mote that is in thy brother's eye, but considerest not the beam that is in thine own eye? Or how wilt thou say to thy brother, Let me pull out the mote out of thine eye; and, behold, a beam is in thine own eye? Thou hypocrite, first cast out the beam out of thine own eye; and then shalt thou see clearly to cast out the mote out of thy brother's eye. Matthew 7:1-5

Obedience is the key. Find out what God's will is for you – and then do what He says.

God Has a Plan

While we can struggle daily in knowing what to do with our lives, God knows our entire destiny. Psalms 139: 16 says, *all the days ordained for me were written in your book before one of them came to me.* (NIV)

It is often difficult to understand the ways of God, he tells us His ways are not our ways. We just have to trust Him.

And as Jesus passed by, he saw a man which was blind from his birth. And his disciples asked him, saying, Master, who did sin, this man, or his parents, that he was born blind? Jesus answered, Neither hath this man sinned, nor his parents: but that the works of God should be made manifest in him. John 9:1-3

God can use illness or a physical situation so that the works of God may be displayed in our life. Many children with asthma "grow out" of the condition as they grow into their teenage years and adulthood. I did not. If I would not have struggled with asthma into my adult years, I would not have been searching for ways to get well and may not have developed an interest in nutrition. It is unlikely that I would have developed a writing career and ultimately, written this book.

Lori wrote:

My friend Melanie was healed from Hodgekin's disease (cancer of the lymph nodes) when she was 13. In 1975, Melanie discovered a lump under her arm and her parents took her to the doctor to find out what it was. The diagnosis was grimm. They diagnosed her with Hodgekin's disease and estimated that she had less than six months to live.

Our church began praying for her as she underwent radiation and chemotherapy. She was very sick from the radiation treatments and lost all her hair from the chemotherapy. To a child of 13 that was very traumatic.

Then, as she progressed, God healed her completely. She told the doctor that God had healed her as she went in for diagnostic tests, and that they weren't going to find anything. They couldn't find any trace of cancer. It was a great testimony to the doctors because they sure didn't expect her to live let alone be completely healed from this cancer.

That was 25 years ago and she is still cancer free and going strong. Today, Melanie is a nurse who often works with cancer patients. Because of her experience, she has great compassion as she knows exactly what they are going through. Most importantly she never forgot that it was God who healed her!

God knows that sometimes in order for us to have true compassion for those around us, we may need to experience what they are going through.

Who comforteth us in all our tribulation, that we may be able to comfort them which are in any trouble, by the comfort wherewith we ourselves are comforted of God. 2 Corinthians 1:4

Be Careful Not to Condemn Others

Remember that it is not always revealed to us why an individual becomes ill. Illness is **NOT ALWAYS** a signal from God that there is unrepented sin, or that it is a punishment for sin, or that they were abusing their bodies in some way. Sometimes we just get sick because we are human with frail physical bodies that get old, break down and are vulnerable to infectious pathogens and toxins in our environment. Our immune systems weaken when we do not take proper care of ourselves – working long hours, not eating enough fruits and vegetables, eating too much sugar, sweets and other refined foods, letting stress get to us, being anxious, not taking enough time to enjoy life, etc. These things do increase our risk of illness, however, sometimes, we just get sick.

The story of Job is probably the best Biblical example we have to demonstrate that not all illness is a consequence of sin. God was actually very angry with Job's three friends as they were convinced that Job's trials were a result of sin against God.

The LORD said to Eliphaz the Temanite, My wrath is kindled against thee, and against thy two friends: for ye have not spoken of me the thing that is right, as my servant Job hath. Job 42:7

Therefore thou art inexcusable, O man, whosoever thou art that judgest: for wherein thou judgest another, thou condemnest thyself; for thou that judgest doest the same things. Romans 2:1

Demonic Forces and Our Health

This is a difficult area to write about. It is not an area I have studied in depth, but what experience I do have has proven to me without a shadow of a doubt that this is a very real problem. Many people choose to be blinded to the fact that demons and demonic possession is a very real problem today, just as it was when Jesus walked the earth.

And the great dragon was cast out, that old serpent, called the Devil, and Satan, which deceiveth the whole world: he was cast out into the earth, and his angels were cast out with him. Revelation 12:9

When Satan was kicked out of heaven, he took one-third of the angels with him (Revelation 12:4). Where do you think all those fallen angels are? They are right here with us on earth – harassing us, tempting us, trying to make our lives miserable any way they can.

When the Bible speaks about Christ healing people of their illnesses, it also lways mentions that He was casting out demons. Many of the sicknesses were caused by demons. Derek Prince, author of the book, *They Shall Expel Demons*, writes, *"One remarkable characteristic of Jesus's ministry, from beginning to end, is that He never made a hard fast distinction between healing people's sickness and delivering them from demons."* He also writes, *"The people who received help from Jesus were mainly normal, respectable, religious people. Yet they were demonized. A demon had gained* access to some area or areas of their personalities and as a result they themselves were not in full control."

One of the first of Jesus's healings mentioned in the Bible is of Simon Peter's mother-in-law.

And he arose out of the synagogue, and entered into Simon's house. And Simon's wife's mother was taken with a great fever; and they besought him for her. And He stood over her, and rebuked the fever; and it left her: and immediately she arose and ministered unto them. Now when the sun was setting, all they that had any sick with divers diseases brought them unto him; and He laid his hands on every one of them, and healed them. And devils also came out of many, crying out, and saying, "Thou art Christ the Son of God." And He rebuking them suffered them not to speak: for they knew that He was Christ. Luke 4:38-41*

How God anointed Jesus of Nazareth with the Holy Ghost and with power: who went about doing good, and healing all that were oppressed of the devil; for God was with him. Acts 10:38*

Many specific health problems are often associated with demonic possession. They include arthritis, epilepsy, alcoholism and addictions, migraines, crippling, blindness, deafness and muteness. It is important to realize that just as all illness is not punishment for sin, all illness is not caused by or related to demonic attack, but we do need to understand that it is a possibility.

Following are a few scriptural references of health problems and demon attack:

Dizziness	Isaiah 19:14
Heaviness/despair	Isaiah 29:10
Blindness	Matthew 12:22
Mute/ robbed of speech	Mark 9:17
Deaf and dumb	Mark 9:25
Infirmity/sickness/crippling	Luke 13:11-13
Incessant pain	2 Corinthians 12:7
Fear	1 Timothy 1:7

And just look at all the problems Satan afflicted Job with: Severe itching (Job 2:8), insomnia (2:4), running sores and scabs (2:5), nightmares (2:12-14), bad breath (19:17), weight loss (19:20), chills and fever (21:6), diarrhea (30:27) and blackened skin (30:30).

Derek Prince compares demonic attack to cancer. *"A human body is regularly attacked by cancerous cells. When the body is healthy, its immune system identifies and attacks the cancerous cells and they are unable to harm the body. But when the body has been weakened by illness or some kind of emotional shock, the immune system is unable to do its job effectively, and some form of cancer can develop somewhere in the body... That's just how it is with demons. Demons continually seek to invade a person, but when the person is healthy spiritually, the spiritual "immune system" within a person identifies and attacks the demons, and they are not able to move in and take control. Any kind of unhealthiness or emotional weakness, on the other hand, makes a person vulnerable to demonic attacks."*

I strongly believe this includes the use of drugs and alcohol, which weaken our defenses. This is discussed later in the book.

In the book of Luke, a woman who is specifically identified as having a "demon of sickness" is healed by Jesus: *And, behold, there was a woman which had a spirit of infirmity eighteen years, and was bowed together, and could in no wise lift up herself. And when Jesus saw her, He called her to him, and said unto her, "Woman, thou art loosed from thine infirmity." And He laid his hands on her: and immediately she was made straight, and glorified God... Satan had bound her for 18 years.* Luke 13:11-13,16

The Bible instructs us how to deal with demonic attack. We must use scripture and the authority we have obtained through the blood of Jesus Christ to cast out demons.

Put on the whole armour of God, that ye may be able to stand against the wiles of the devil. For we wrestle not against flesh and blood, but against principalities, against powers, against the rulers of the darkness of this world, against spiritual wickedness in high places. Ephesians 6:11-12

And when He had called unto Him his twelve disciples, He gave them power (and authority) against unclean spirits, to cast them out, and to heal (cure) all manner of sickness and all manner of disease, (weakness and infirmity). Matthew 10:1-2, (Parenthesis are added from the Amplified Bible)

37

These twelve Jesus sent forth, and commanded them, saying, Go not into the way of the Gentiles, and into any city of the Samaritans enter ye not: But go rather to the lost sheep of the house of Israel. And as ye go, preach, saying, The kingdom of heaven is at hand. Heal the sick, cleanse the lepers, raise the dead, cast out devils: freely ye have received, freely give. Matthew 10:5-8

Howard wrote:

I have had a problem with acid-reflux for some time. It really bothered me at night when I laid down to go to sleep and would keep me up at night. It was especially bad if I ate spicy food.

I was reading "The Bondage Breaker" by Neil Anderson and was learning about the possibility of demonic influences that could be causing or contributing to the problem. One time when I was having the problem, I decided to rebuke that spirit and sure enough the pain went away. It has come back since then, but every time it does, I rebuke that spirit in the name of Jesus and it gets better.

If you want to learn more about this area, a good place to start is by reading *They Shall Expel Demons* by Derek Prince.

Additional causes of sickness are covered later.

The First Sin... Food and Obedience

I thought it interesting that the first sin involved food. In the book of Genesis, God gave Adam and Eve all the fruit to eat, except the fruit of the tree of knowledge of good and evil, under the Noahic covenant. In Genesis 8 and 9:3, God adds animals to the list of food for man. Bread is symbolic of Christ [John 6 and 1Corinthians 11:24]. Natural food is for the natural man and spiritual food is for the spiritual man. Food often represents the appetites of the natural man. Appetites of this nature can carry us away from God (feeding our flesh - gluttony, etc.). When we control our appetites as such, we will draw nearer to God, for example, in fasting.

God intended food to be good for man, but sin in man corrupted even that. This sin caused some changes in man as well – our natural bodies do not live forever, although that was how God had originally designed them. We must dwell in our corrupted bodies, but God can heal and restore them and promises a new spiritual body. We are not to set our affections on foods, but instead on God, as we struggle with our appetites day by day. The goal is to hold back on our desires from the natural man and feed our spiritual man.

God Wants Us to Seek Him

Seek the LORD and his strength, seek his face continually. 1Chronicles 16:11

But seek ye first the kingdom of God, and his righteousness; and all these things shall be added unto you. Matthew 6:33

When we put God's kingdom first, He will take care of everything else! Whenever you have a problem or are in trouble (or better yet, *before* you are in trouble) ask yourself: am I seeking the Kingdom of God first or am I concerned more about my physical needs? Ask yourself: is my physical or financial well-being worthy of such devotion in my life? If you think it is, then your god is mammon, your life is cursed with worry, and you live life concerned mostly with physical needs. If you do not think that your physical well being is a worthy object to live your life for, you then may enjoy heavenly treasure, rest in divine provision, and fulfill God's highest purpose for ourself: fellowship with Him, and being part of His kingdom. We need to keep our priorities in order. We need to focus on God and not on our physical weaknesses.

Remember, this is the choice that you made when you became a Christian; but at that time, many of us did not realize the full significance of its meaning. This is what spiritual growth is all about. This decision needs to be reinforced everyday of your life.

Peter reminds us of the importance of being useful and productive in knowing Christ. This is the end to which we have died to ourselves and now live for Jesus Christ. Peter defines this as having faith, goodness, knowledge, self-control, perseverance, godliness, brotherly kindness and love.

Second Peter 1:5-7 tells us that as we advance toward our goal of knowing Christ more each day, these qualities will advance in us.

How do you gauge your growth in Christ? Ask the Great Physician for a spiritual check-up. Once you have trusted Him as your personal Savior, you are provided with everything you need to grow in your relationship with Him. God accepts you just as you are, *but His heart's desire is to move you from where you are to where He is* (Hebrews 10:14).

Spiritual growth does not just happen: *Therefore, I will always be ready to remind you of these things, even though you already know them, and have been established in the truth which is present with you* (2 Peter 1:12).

In your spiritual check-up, ask Jesus:

- Have I allowed false teachers to deceive me?

- Am I getting caught up in physical, material and worldly things that will eventually all turn to ashes?

- Are my priorities in the right order?

- Am I trusting God with my whole life or am I holding onto certain things?

- Am I "letting You do it" or am I trying to do things myself?

He will show you which areas of your life are inhibiting your growth. The wonder of the Great Physician is that He never shows you what needs healing without giving you the right prescription for change and healing: *And you shall know the truth and the truth shall make you free* (John 8:32).

If you are truly seeking God, but there is an area in your life that is interfering with your relationship with Him, this is the area He is likely to test you on. For example, several times the Bible warns us that personal gain and finances will interfere with our relationship with God.

Then Jesus, beholding him, loved him, and said unto him, One thing thou lackest: go thy way, sell whatsoever thou hast, and give to the poor, and thou shalt have treasure in heaven: and come, take up the cross, and follow me. And he was sad at that saying, and went away grieved: for he had great possessions. And Jesus looked round about, and saith unto his disciples, How hardly shall they that have riches enter into the kingdom of God! And the disciples were astonished at his words. But Jesus answereth again, and saith unto them, Children, how hard is it for them that trust in riches to enter into the kingdom of God! It is easier for a camel to go through the eye of a needle, than for a rich man to enter into the kingdom of God. Mark 10:21-25

It is very true. If God told you to sell everything that you have, give the money to the poor, and follow Him, would you? How many people do you know who would be willing to make that sacrifice? *For where your treasure is, there will your heart be also* (Matthew 6:21). What are some of the other things we put before God?

1. Self (personal problems, health, our circumstances, etc.) - It's not about you!

2. Spouse or personal relationships

3. Work

4. Personal gain or social status

5. Family

Anything in your life that becomes more important than God and your relationship with Him becomes a form of idolatry. Don't forget, this is the very first commandment - *Thou shalt have no other gods before me* (Exodus 20:3).

If we are not seeking Him, if God is not **first** in our lives, if we are not willing to give up everything for him, He will still seek us just as a shepherd will leave the herd to find a lost sheep.

For the Son of man is come to save that which was lost. How think ye? if a man have an hundred sheep, and one of them be gone astray, doth he not leave the ninety and nine, and goeth into the mountains, and seeketh that which is gone astray? And if so be that he find it, verily I say unto you, he rejoiceth more of that sheep, than of the ninety and nine which went not astray. Even so it is not the will of your Father which is in heaven, that one of these little ones should perish. Moreover, if thy brother shall trespass against thee, go and tell him his fault between thee and him alone: if he shall hear thee, thou hast gained thy brother. But if he will not hear thee, then take with thee one or two more, that in the mouth of two or three witnesses every word may be established. And if he shall neglect to hear them, tell it unto the church: but if he neglect to hear the church, let him be unto thee as an heathen man and a publican. Verily I say unto you, Whatsoever ye shall bind on earth shall be bound in heaven: and whatsoever ye shall loose on earth shall be loosed in heaven. Matthew 18:11-18

Gail wrote:

I've always claimed that my Multiple Sclerosis was a gift from God at a time in my life that was crucial considering all the things that have gone on since. I believe it was His way of slowing me down to appreciate the things around me that I was rushing by. It woke me up to reality and what is really important in life.

I have since endured the loss of my mother, a

son who is in prison, and breast cancer resulting in a mastectomy. Through it all, I knew my Savior was right by my side to catch me when I'd fall and carry me till I could walk on my own again. I know now that my M S was His wake up call for me, and I am so grateful for that. God is good... All the time!

A Test of Faith

When God tests our faith and we are faced with trials, it is often more difficult to understand, especially in the midst of the suffering. Job lost all his livestock, his fruit trees, his family and his friends. Then, he was afflicted with painful boils all over his body. *So went Satan forth from the presence of the LORD, and smote Job with sore boils from the sole of his foot unto his crown* (Job 2:7). Job searched his heart to see if there was unconfessed sin and could find none.

But may the God of all grace, who called us to His eternal glory by Christ Jesus . . . perfect, establish, strengthen, and settle you. 1 Peter 5:10

In order to perfect our lives, God needs to strengthen us, to develop our lives spiritually, so that we can grow closer to him. To do this, we will have to go through trials and the useful (though often undesired) suffering that is required.

Suffering is often the link between the work God wants to do in us and the abundant grace that He will use to effect the work: *after you have suffered a while.*

Even as the perfect, sinless man, the Son of God learned valuable lessons through suffering. *Though He was a Son, yet He learned obedience by the things which He suffered* (Hebrews 5:8). He experienced the agonies that can be involved in obeying God while dwelling in a rebellious, sinful world.

Such trials and sufferings are normal and purposeful. *Beloved, do not think it strange concerning the fiery trial which is to try you, as though some strange thing happened to you* (1 Peter 4:12). Painful trials may seem strange – even cruel. We may feel like we are the only one who has ever suffered so greatly and question, "Why me, God?" as if we are perfect, are always in the perfect will of God and our relationship with Him is perfect. Trials routinely come to test and exercise our faith. God knows our heart and only He knows what it will take in order to humble us, challenge us and mature us.

And thou shalt remember all the way which the LORD thy God led thee these forty years in the wilderness, to humble thee, and to prove thee, to know what was in thine heart, whether thou wouldest keep his commandments, or no. And he humbled thee, and suffered thee to hunger, and fed thee with manna, which thou knewest not, neither did thy fathers know; that he might make thee know that man doth not live by bread only, but by every word that proceedeth out of the mouth of the LORD doth man live. Deuteronomy 8:2-3

And whosoever shall exalt himself shall be abased; and he that shall humble himself shall be exalted. Matthew 23:12

But he giveth more grace. Wherefore he saith, God resisteth the proud, but giveth grace unto the humble. James 4:6

When we are humbled by God (which can be quite an experience in itself), He can finally give us His grace. Trials and suffering humble us and stir us to cry out to the Lord for His necessary grace. In Paul's most persistent trial of suffering, he said, *Lest I should be exalted above measure by the abundance of the revelations, a thorn in the flesh was given to me . . . Concerning this thing I pleaded with the Lord three times that it might depart from me* (2 Corinthians 12:7-8). That's exactly what God wants. He wants us to acknowledge the fact that we need Him – to earnestly plead with Him with a contrite heart. The Lord responded by His grace. And He said to me, *My grace is sufficient for you, for My strength is made perfect in weakness. Therefore most gladly I will rather boast in my infirmities, that the power of Christ may rest upon me* (2 Corinthians 12:9). Paul did not receive the healing grace that he sought. However, he experienced the sustaining grace that God often chooses to impart in times of suffering. Through His grace, God changed Paul's heart, not his circumstances.

How often when we are going through a trial do we pray that God will change our circumstances rather than change our heart (to rely upon Him) so we can deal with the circumstances or to have insight into what God is trying to teach us? During the sufferings and trials, we need to take the focus off of ourselves, and place it where it belongs – on Him.

Growing Pains

God told Jeremiah to go down to the potter's house and learn a valuable lesson about life. (Jeremiah 18:1-6) Jeremiah watched the potter working the wheel. The potter would gather a shapeless mass of clay, plop it on the wheel and begin turning the wheel by pumping a pedal with his foot. As the wheel turned, the potter shaped and squeezed the lump of clay into a graceful shape. If the potter didn't like the result, he'd simply start again. He would dampen the clay and begin to mold it into an entirely different object. He might turn a low, wide cooking bowl into a slim, tall drinking jar. The potter would keep trying until he got exactly the shape and size vessel he wanted.

God treats us as clay just like the potter. He molds us into different shapes and sizes. He works some into plain looking bowls and others into elaborate vases. Sometimes He doesn't like what he sees, so He scoops up the clay and starts again.

This is a wonderful and reassuring lesson about our lives. God isn't through with us when things go wrong, when we become flawed by failure or misshapen by events. God is determined to make something beautiful and useful out of our lives, no matter how long it takes, no matter how much we resist Him.

I heard a beautiful version about Jeremiah's lesson at a women's retreat a few years back. While the woman spoke, she was sitting at a potter's wheel demonstrating, giving us a wonderful visual. As she worked the clay she explained how the clay usually has ideas of "her" own and may not always cooperate with the potter. The clay complained and cried out in pain as the potter didn't like how the clay was turning out so she had to smash the clay down and start over. This happened many times until the clay finally conceded and cooperated. The clay finally got tired of "getting beat up" and let the potter do what she wanted. The clay was still complaining when the potter made it into a large wide bowl. The clay didn't want to be a bowl, it wanted to be a tall, thin elegant vase maybe to hold flowers.

When the potter was done shaping the bowl it had to be trimmed and shaved. The clay complained the whole time, "That hurts. Ouch. Be careful. Why are you doing that to me? Is this really necessary?"

When finished, the potter uprooted the clay from its comfortable base (again to the great discomfort of the clay) and put the bowl into the hot oven to be fired. The clay especially did not like that. When the bowl came out, still complaining, the potter then sat the bowl on a shelf. The bowl cried, "First you make me into a stupid bowl and now you just have me sittin' here on the shelf. What good am I doing here?"

The bowl sat and sat. Months went by, and then years. Finally, one day the potter took the bowl and sent it out. That bowl was then used to hold the water to wash the dirty, tired feet of a man named Jesus.

Do You Trust God?

We all have things we need to deal with – or that God wants us to deal with. It is important not to try to stuff these issues and pretend they don't exist – past sin, emotional trauma from abuse, neglect, abandonment, etc. If we try to hold on to things (pain) that God wants us to turn over to Him, He will likely not let us have peace until we do.

We can rejoice in the fact that we grow spiritually as He sees us through our trials. Sometimes it is hard to believe that God really loves us or really forgives us. We think, "but I have a lot of sin to be forgiven for." *But where sin abounded, grace did much more abound* (Romans 5:20).

We need this grace, because this may be a place of great vulnerability where Satan will try to harass us. He will try to make us feel unworthy and rejected over past mistakes, and fearful that we will make mistakes in the future. We must trust God. We must believe His promises. We must stop beating ourselves up. If we were beaten or robbed every time we walked down a certain street, would we continue going down that same street? I hope not!

We should take great comfort in knowing that God has a plan for us. If we are willing to trust him and let Him have complete control over our lives, not only can He use us, but He can bless us.

When Jesus was at the synagogue he said to a man with a shrivelled hand: *Stretch forth thine hand. And he stretched it forth; and it was restored whole, like as the other* (Matthew 12:10-13).

The fact that Jesus instructed the man to stretch out his hand shows there was a connection between faith and healing power. God does not just do every-thing for us automatically. There may be a "test" – "a crisis of belief" requiring action on our part.

God may convict you to quit smoking, or to stop drinking so much pop or coffee or eating so much sugar, or meat, or eating so much period! He may con-vict you to correct your eating habits before He will heal your diabetes or high blood pressure or arthritis. If He is, this is what you need to do to be healed. If He tells you that you have headaches or a rash or a tumor because of a sin in your life, and that if you repent from your sin that you will be healed, you must take action so God will bless you.

If you are suffering from a chronic health problem and want to be healed, you must spend time with God and find out if there is anything He wants to tell you. If you humbly pray, He will reveal it.

Then Jeremiah the prophet said unto them, I have heard [you]; behold, I will pray unto the LORD your God according to your words; and it shall come to pass, [that] whatsoever thing the LORD shall answer you, I will declare [it] unto you; I will keep nothing back from you. Jeremiah 42:4

The revelation may not come right at the time you are praying, so you need to be ready (and listening). Maybe the Holy Spirit will convict you the next time you pick up a donut to eat for breakfast. Maybe the person you need to forgive will call you right out of the blue and the Holy Spirit will convict you. There will be no flashing blue lights. This is not KMart. God's ways are not our ways. Usually, God will speak with subtlety. Every time God speaks to us it will test our faith and we will ask, "Is that you God?" Until we *know* it is him. This is part of the growth process.

And when he putteth forth his own sheep, he goeth before them, and the sheep follow him: for they know his voice. John 10:4

Remember, whenever you ask God for something, to pay attention to what happens the next few days or weeks. Don't just forget about it. He wants us to be in constant communion with Him. How can we get the answer if we are not listening? How would you feel if you got a phone call from someone you loved dearly and they spent 10 or 15 minutes telling you all about their problems, asking you a lot of questions (which you had all the answers for), listing a bunch of requests for other people you also cared deeply about and then they simply hung up? When you called them back to try to comfort them and give them their answers, they were too busy doing their own thing to even answer the phone.

This is often how we treat God. We talk to God when it is convenient for us. We pray, but don't bother to pick up a Bible. God has many answers for us right there in that amazing book, but you have to pick it up and open it. He answers us in many other ways too, but we have to truly be seeking Him and His will.

A Letter:

As you got up this morning, I watched you, and hoped you would talk to me, even if it was just a few words, asking my opinion or thanking me for something good that happened in your life yesterday. But I noticed you were too busy, trying to find the right outfit to wear. When you ran around the house getting ready, I knew there would be a few minutes for you to stop and say hello, but you were too busy.

At one point you had to wait 15 minutes with nothing to do except sit in a chair. Then I saw you spring to your feet. I thought you wanted to talk to me but you ran to the phone and called a friend instead. I watched patiently all day long.

With all your activities I guess you were too busy to say anything to me. I noticed that before lunch you looked around, maybe you felt embarrassed to talk to me, that is why you didn't bow your head. You glanced three or four tables over and you noticed some of your friends talking to me briefly before they ate, but you didn't. That's okay. There is still more time left, and I hope that you will talk to me yet. You went home and it seems as if you had lots of things to do.

After a few of them were done, you turned on the TV. I don't know if you like TV or not, just about anything goes there and you spend a lot of time each day in front of it not thinking about anything, just enjoying the show. I waited patiently again as you watched the TV and ate your meal, but again you didn't talk to me.

At bedtime I guess you felt too tired. After you said goodnight to your family, you plopped into bed and fell asleep in no time. That's okay because you may not realize that I am always there for you. I've got patience, more than you will ever know.

I even want to teach you how to be patient with others as well. I love you so much that I wait every-day for a nod, prayer or thought or a thankful part of your heart. It is hard to have a one-sided conver-sation. Well, you are getting up once again. And once again I will wait, with nothing but love for you. Hoping that today you will give me some time.

Have a nice day!

Love, GOD

I know several times I have prayed asking for something and have just about missed the answer. God does not always answer our prayers in the way that we expect and He often does not answer our prayers immediately. It may be the next day or the next week. It just shows me how important it is to pay attention to what God is trying to tell us at <u>all times</u> – to be in con-stant communion with Him. I wonder how many times I have missed the answer because I was so wrapped up in what I thought was important.

God definitely does speak to us through the scrip-tures, so we must spend time in the Word – everyday. Many times I have opened my Bible right to a scripture that addressed the exact situation I was praying about. But if I had not opened my Bible after praying, God never would have been able to communicate with me what He wanted to tell me. God does answer our prayers. We simply must do our part by listening for the answer.

Obedience

And why call ye me, Lord, Lord, and do not the things which I say? Luke 6:46

After we get an answer to prayer, the next step is to obey. If God prompts you to eat a healthy diet so that He will cleanse your arteries of the plaque and debris that is inhibiting optimal blood flow to your heart and throughout your body, you had better listen. In obedience, you start eating whole grain foods high in cleansing fiber, fruits and vegetables rich in healing phytochemicals, cut back on meat, not eating the fat and increase healthier sources of protein such as fish, cut back on sugar and processed foods, etc. God is faithful and He will heal you. But if, after a time, you decide to return to your old eating habits, what do you think will happen? We cannot continue to do what got us sick in the first place and expect to be healed or remain healed.

Jesus healed a man who had been lame for 38 years at the pools in Bethesda telling him to pick up his bed and walk. Notice the action required through faith by the man (John 5:8). *Afterward, Jesus findeth him in the temple, and said unto him, Behold, thou art made whole: sin no more, <u>lest a worse thing come unto thee</u>* (John 5:14).

We must repent. We cannot continue doing what

we are doing and expect God to bless us. That is not how He works.

But without faith it is impossible to please Him: for he that cometh to God must believe that He is, and that He is a rewarder of them that diligently seek Him. Hebrews 11:6

Trials force us to look beyond what is in our own strength and ability. We agonize over our situation trying to figure out why such a thing has happened. This is exactly what God wants. Some people choose to simply ignore the situation that God has presented or is allowing us to go through. Many people busy themselves in work, community or other activities waiting for the situation to go away. Other people often choose to turn to pain pills, sleeping pills, antidepressants, other drugs or alcohol to help them run away from the problem. These do not not allow us to grow in the grace of God. They hinder our relationship with Him. You can't run away from God!

Our biggest obstacle is usually fear – not trusting God. We think we need to be in control instead of just letting go and letting God do it.

If life were easy, what would we need God for? He wants us to need Him, to seek Him. He wants us to TOTALLY RELY ON HIM – that's the whole point. If we don't, we can't grow in Him. Why do you think the Bible instructs us so many times to "be strong and of good courage"? (28 times, by the way)

Have not I commanded thee? Be strong and of a good courage; be not afraid, neither be thou dis-

mayed: for the LORD thy God is with thee whither-
soever thou goest. Joshua 1:9

God is our refuge and strength, a very present
help in trouble. Psalms 46:1

O my soul, don't be discouraged. Don't be
upset. Expect God to act! For I know that I shall
again have plenty of reason to praise Him for all
that He will do. He is my help! He is my God! Psalm
42:11

Pray without ceasing. In everything give
thanks: for this is the will of God in Jesus Christ
concerning you. 1 Thessalonians 5:17-18

Betty wrote:

When I was three months away from 16 years
of age, I had my first son, Kevin. He died at birth. At
that time I did not know Jesus as my Lord. My hus-
band, who knew God, wrote in the book from the
funeral home, something the preacher had said in
the funeral message (I didn't remember any of it):
"David said, 'My son can't come back to be with me
but I can go to be with him.'" When I read that, I
thought that was what I wanted to do. The next
Sunday, November of 1964, I went to church with
my mother-in-law and I accepted Jesus into my
heart and I have never regretted it. He is as real to
me now as He was then and has never let me down.
I lost three more babies in miscarriages after that

but He saw me through. I finally told God that if He would give me a baby and let it live, I would raise it for Him. He not only gave me one, He gave me a son and then a daughter. They are now 30 and 33 years old. I did my best to raise them for God and they love God. What a wonderful friend Jesus has been to me.

Gini wrote:

There was a morning that I just couldn't get out of bed – to deal with three children and a demanding husband – let alone a three-story house. My left thumb was terribly swollen, sore, and paining. Arthritis, of course. I prayed right then, "God, I have this job to do. Since my children are adopted, (a blessing I had prayed for), I assume you want me to take good care of them. You know how difficult they are. I need your help to get out of this bed and do my job. This thumb needs your attention badly. I am not asking you to take away everything; but I am asking for the energy for the day and the relief for my thumb." I was able after a few moments to get up; relief came for my thumb. However, it remained swollen and has a knot on it to this day. The message I received was that it wouldn't be easy, but I would be able to continue. I wondered whether I had been "hard" on God, too direct; but I knew he was well aware of all my situation. My thumb remains a constant reminder to me that I would remain able to continue.

God Is On Our Side

The only survivor of a shipwreck was washed up on a small, uninhabited island. He prayed fervently for God to rescue him and everyday he scanned the horizon for help but none seemed forthcoming. Exhausted, he eventually managed to build a little hut out of driftwood to protect him from the elements, and to store his few possessions. But then one day, after scavenging for food, he arrived home to find his little hut in flames, the smoke rolling up to the sky. The worst had happened; everything was lost. He was stunned with grief and anger. "God, how could you do this to me!" he cried.

Early the next day, however, he was awakened by the sound of a ship that was approaching the island. It had come to rescue him. "How did you know I was here?" asked the weary man of his rescuers.

"We saw your smoke signal," they replied.

It is easy to get discouraged when things are going bad. But we shouldn't lose heart, because God is at work in our lives, even in the midst of pain and suffering. Remember, next time your little hut is burning to the ground, it just may be a smoke signal that summons the grace of God.

For all the negative things we have to say to ourselves, God has a positive answer for it:

You say: It's impossible.
God says: All things are possible. Luke 18:27

You say: I'm too tired.
God says: I will give you rest. Matthew 11:28-30
You say: Nobody really loves me.

God says: I love you. John 3:16 and John 13:34

You say: I can't go on.
God says: My grace is sufficient. 2 Corinthians 12:9

You say: I can't figure things out.
God says: I will direct your steps. Proverbs 3.5-6

You say: I can't do it.
God says: You can do all things. Phillipians 4:13

You say: I'm not able.
God says: I am able. 2 Corinthians 9:8

You say: It's not worth it.
God says: It will be worth it. Roman 8:28

You say: I can't forgive myself.
God says: I forgive you. I John 1:9 and Romans 8:1

You say: I can't manage.
God says: I will supply all your needs. Phillipians 4:19

You say: I'm afraid.
God says: I have not given you a spirit of fear.
2 Timothy 1:7

You say: I'm always worried and frustrated.
God says: Cast all your cares on ME. 1 Peter 5:7

You say: I don't have enough faith.
God says: I've given everyone the measure of faith.
Romans 12:3

You say: I'm not smart enough.
God says: I give you wisdom. 1Corinthians 1:30

You say: I feel all alone.
God says: I will never leave you nor forsake you. Hebrews 13:5

With God on our side, how can anything go wrong?

Does God Really Heal People Today?

Why wouldn't God heal people today? It would be like saying, "well, some of the Bible applies to today, but not all of it."

The prophets also had the ability to heal. This was perhaps to show people the character of God. He used the prophets to demonstrate his love and concern for each of us.

Luke, a physician himself, wrote extensively about the healing ministry of Jesus because He had great compassion for the sick, the weak, the poor.

And He (Jesus) came down with them, and stood in the plain, and the company of His disciples, and a great multitude of people out of all Judea and Jerusalem, and from the sea coast of Tyre and Sidon, which came to hear Him, and to be healed of their diseases; And they that were vexed with unclean spirits: and they were healed. And the whole multitude sought to touch him: for there went virtue out of Him, and healed them all. And He lifted up his eyes on his disciples, and said, Blessed be ye poor: for yours is the kingdom of God. Blessed are ye that hunger now: for ye shall be filled. Blessed are ye that weep now: for ye shall laugh. Blessed are ye, when men shall hate you, and when they shall separate you from their company, and shall reproach you, and cast out your name as evil, for the Son of man's sake. Rejoice ye in that day, and leap for joy: for, behold, your reward is great in heaven: for in the like manner did their fathers unto the prophets. Luke 6:17-23

Jesus healed people when He was here to show his character. He healed people to show He was God. Healing was also a visable affirmation of His ability to forgive sin. (Luke 5:24) We all have sin, we all need to be healed.

He performed "miracles" for the people because in our "humanness" it is hard to believe without some sort of miraculous demonstration. Most of the miracles He performed involved helping of those in need by healing and providing food (Feeding the 5,000 – Luke 9:16), Feeding the 4,000 – Mark 8:1-9). God is very concerned about our physical needs.

People travelled from all over (without cars or modern transportation) to be healed. Jesus must have had an awesome presence about Him. Just at the sight of Him people would bow down and worship.

And it came to pass, when He was in a certain city, behold a man full of leprosy: who seeing Jesus fell on His face, and besought him, saying, Lord, if thou wilt, thou canst make me clean. Luke 5:12

And, behold, there cometh one of the rulers of the synagogue, Jairus by name; and when he saw Him, he fell at his feet, And besought him greatly, saying, My little daughter lieth at the point of death: I pray thee, come and lay thy hands on her, that she may be healed; and she shall live. And Jesus went with him; and much people followed him, and thronged Him. Mark 5:22 -23

In the meantime, a ruler from inside the synagogue informed them, *Thy daughter is dead: why troublest thou the Master any further? When Jesus heard this, He saith unto the ruler of the synagogue, Be not afraid, only believe. They went to the house where the young girl lay dead. When they arrived everyone was weeping and grieving. Jesus said, Why make ye this ado, and weep? the damsel is not dead, but sleepeth* (Mark 5:40).

The people all laughed at Him. He took the mother and father of the child to where she was lying.

And He took the damsel by the hand, and said unto her, Talitha cumi; which is, being interpreted, Damsel, I say unto thee, arise. And straightway the damsel arose, and walked; for she was of the age of twelve years. And they were astonished with a great astonishment. And He charged them straitly that no man should know it; and commanded that something should be given her to eat. Mark 5:41-43

Before they had gone to the house, another incident occurred:

And a certain woman, which had an issue of

blood twelve years, And had suffered many things of many physicians, and had spent all that she had, and was nothing bettered, but rather grew worse, When she had heard of Jesus, came in the press behind, and touched his garment. For she said, If I may touch but His clothes, I shall be whole. And straightway the fountain of her blood was dried up; and she felt in her body that she was healed of that plague. And Jesus, immediately knowing in Himself that virtue had gone out of Him, turned Him about in the press, and said, Who touched my clothes? And His disciples said unto Him, Thou seest the multitude thronging thee, and sayest thou, Who touched me? And He looked round about to see her that had done this thing. But the woman fearing and trembling, knowing what was done in her, came and fell down before Him, and told him all the truth. And He said unto her, Daughter, thy faith hath made thee whole; go in peace, and be whole of thy plague.
Mark 5:25-34

This story also makes an interesting point about something that is very common today: *And had suffered many things of many physicians,* **and had spent all that she had**, *and was nothing bettered, but rather grew worse.* She had gone to one physician after another trying everything, spending all her money in attempt to get well. Isn't that what most of us do? Go to one doctor after another, try one prescription after another, one supplement after another? Yet nothing works. Why? Often we look everywhere for help but where God wants us to look – to Him. He is the Great Physician.

Also note that this woman had so much faith that she believed that she only had to touch his clothes and that she would be made whole. Where is our faith? When you pray for healing, do you believe **without a doubt** that God can heal you? Jesus also told the ruler of the synagogue, ***Be not afraid, only believe*** when they were informed of his daughter's death. Where is our faith today?

And ye shall serve the LORD your God, and He shall bless thy bread, and thy water; and I will take sickness away from the midst of thee. Exodus 23: 25-26

Bless the LORD, O my soul, and forget not all his benefits: Who forgiveth all thine iniquities; who healeth all thy diseases; Psalm 103:2-3

For I will restore health unto thee, and I will heal thee of thy wounds, saith the LORD. Jeremiah 30:17

Jesus is the Great Physician

Jesus healed a crippled man by the Bethesda pools in Jerusalem.

And a certain man was there, who had been thirty and eight years in his infirmity. When Jesus saw him lying, and knew that he had been now a long time in that case, He saith unto him, Wouldest thou be made whole? The sick man answered him, Sir, I have no man, when the water is troubled, to put me into the pool: but while I am coming, another steppeth down before me. Jesus saith unto him, Arise, take up thy bed, and walk. And straightway the man was made whole, and took up his bed and walked. John 5:5-9

Muriel wrote:

I was diagnosed with multiple sclerosis at the age of 24, both at the Mayo Clinic and the Fargo Neurological Institute. I had double vision, blindness in one eye and a weak right leg, etc. These symptoms came and went, which is typical of this disease. There was a travelling evangelistic who came to our church in 1973 and he prayed for people. I went forward for prayer and felt absolutely nothing and was so disappointed. Then I went to bed that night and my body became alive with electricity. It continued for several hours. I was healed and have had no problems with M.S. since. The doctors say that I must be in remission, but I know that God has healed me. This has led me to search for God in a deeper way than I had never known before and continues to this day. It changed my life completely. I saw Him as a God of miracles that I knew nothing about. I knew that there was so much more to this "Christian" life to learn and experience. It has been great!

Judy wrote:

I was having a lot of pain in my female organs for about a month and was taking Ibuprofen for the pain. I was told by a doctor to discontinue taking the 3,200 mg. a day as it could do kidney damage. They recommended a hysterectomy. At that time, we were having small group meetings for Bible study and prayer weekly in our home, so I took the problem to our group and asked for prayer. They laid hands on me and asked for healing. That was 12 years ago, and everything is still in tact and working well. Praise God.

Judy continues:

I found my Mom in a lot of pain one morning at my sister's house. I called my other sister who was Inservice Director at the LaPalma Hospital. She told me to have her brought there by ambulance and she'd have a doctor waiting for her in the ER. We got her there, and the tests started. They first gave her a shot to raise her low blood pressure. She screamed and grabbed her head. My brother, sister and I went immediately to the chapel and fell on our knees. I asked the Lord to watch over her and protect her for fear of the incompetency of the doctors care she was under.

They took x-rays, had someone read them, but couldn't find anything. They couldn't give her a shot or any medication for pain until they found out what was wrong. It just so happened my uncle (a radiologist) was visiting us from Loma Linda. He went in and asked if he could look at the x-rays. He detected a slight shadow and said he thought she was passing some small gravel-like stones from her gall bladder surgery that was performed a week or so before that. He deducted her bile ducts hadn't been cleaned out thoroughly.

They took her into ICU and put the tubes down her throat and said they still couldn't give her anything for pain, which she was in a lot of. I was standing by her bedside watching her when I noticed blood in her tube. I called my sister (who was the Inservice Director) over and asked if that was normal. She insisted they had put the tube down her lungs, so the nurses had to reinsert the tube. At this point I was so frustrated, frightened and disgusted with hospital care, I laid hands on her and prayed. I said that I had the faith to ask, believe and claim healing in my mother's stead and I thanked God for healing her. This was at 9:30 p.m. I went home resting assuredly that she was going to be O.K.

The next morning I was informed that everything broke loose around 2:30 a.m. and that my mother started feeling better. By 6:00 a.m. she wanted to get up and told them she was ready to go home. They put her in a room and said she'd have to wait. By the time I got back there around 8:00 a.m. she was eating breakfast and the attending doctor came in to check her. The doctor said, "I don't understand this at all. What has happened here?" I told her we had called on the Great Physician to heal her. She was very uncomfortable with that statement and quickly wrote her notes on the chart and left the room. I then told Mom that I had prayed for her the previous night. Tears welled up in her eyes and we thanked the Lord for His graciousness.

Melvin said:

I had taken a week's vacation off of work in the fall in order to cut wood to heat the house for my family for the winter. I was out chopping wood and suddenly my back went out. Normally, when that happens I would be out of commission for at least a week. I knew it was bad because I could feel the tingling (from probably a pinched sciatic nerve) all the way down my leg. I called my wife and kids to all pray for me because I knew the Lord could heal me. They laid hands on me and prayed and just like that my back was fine. I went back to chopping and worked the rest of the week.

Anything is possible if you have faith. Mark 9:23

There is Only One Healer

There are individuals who have been given the gift of healing, but they are not the ones doing the healing. God has chosen them as servants to do His work.

Healing can be a great ministry, but the glory must be given to God and reverence must be maintained as holy worship should be. It is so irritating to watch such disrespectful situations on television or elsewhere that do not present this requirement. If the glory does not go to God – turn the channel.

God heals who He wants, and when He wants. These individuals cannot heal whoever they want to heal. Don't believe false promises or guarantees to be healed. In these situations one needs to be very careful.

In Matthew we see an example of Jesus healing on the premise of belief:

And, behold, a woman, which was diseased with an issue of blood twelve years, came behind Him, and touched the hem of his garment: For she said within herself, If I may but touch his garment, I shall be whole. But Jesus turned him about, and when He saw her, He said, Daughter, be of good comfort; thy faith hath made thee whole. And the woman was made whole from that hour. Matthew 9:20-22

Sometimes the sick were healed so that others would see and believe.

And, behold, they brought to Him a man sick of the palsy, lying on a bed: and Jesus seeing their faith said unto the sick of the palsy; Son, be of good cheer; thy sins be forgiven thee. And, behold, certain of the scribes said within themselves, This man blasphemeth. And Jesus knowing their thoughts said, Wherefore think ye evil in your hearts? For whether is easier, to say, Thy sins be forgiven thee;

or to say, Arise, and walk? But that ye may know that the Son of man hath power on earth to forgive sins, (then saith he to the sick of the palsy,) Arise, take up thy bed, and go unto thine house. And he arose, and departed to his house. But when the multitudes saw it, they marvelled, and glorified God, which had given such power unto men. Matthew 9:2-8

Healings by Jesus or the disciples brought many, many people to beleive in the Lord. *They brought forth the sick into the streets, and laid them on beds and couches, that at the least the shadow of Peter passing by might overshadow some of them. There came also a multitude out of the cities round about unto Jerusalem, bringing sick folks, and them which were vexed with unclean spirits: and they were healed every one* (Acts 5:14-16).

If you are not healed, it does not necessarily mean that you did not believe. If you have gone to a healer or to the elders of the church or had people pray over you for healing, but you are not healed, there may be several reasons. Here are some to think about:

1. God may want you to deal with unconfessed sin.

In order to be forgiven (and blessed) we need to confess our sin and repent from it. *Who forgiveth all thine iniquities; who healeth all thy diseases* (Psalm 103:3).

You may have personal habits or obsessions that

you are still holding onto which God wants you to release. You may be harboring anger or hurt feeling towards someone. He may want you to let go and forgive them. *For if ye forgive men their trespasses, your heavenly Father will also forgive you: But if ye forgive not men their trespasses, neither will your Father forgive your trespasses* (Matthew 6:14-15)

In Paul's first letter to the Corinthians, He makes it very clear that we need to examine ourselves for unrepented sin in our lives before we can receive His full blessing and to partake in Holy Communion. Sickness and death are specified as disciplinary actions for our sin.

But let a man examine himself, and so let him eat of that bread, and drink of that cup. For he that eateth and drinketh unworthily, eateth and drinketh damnation to himself, not discerning the Lord's body. For this cause many are weak and sickly among you, and many sleep. For if we would judge ourselves, we should not be judged. But when we are judged, we are chastened of the Lord, that we should not be condemned with the world. 1Corinthians 11:28-32

2. God may be dissatisfied with your service to Him.

With faith, simple belief is inadequate. With belief comes the responsibility to do the will of the Father - including service to mankind. This service must also be done with the right heart.

What doth it profit, my brethren, though a man say he hath faith, and have not works? Can faith save him? If a brother or sister be naked, and destitute of daily food, And one of you say unto them, Depart in peace, be ye warmed and filled; notwithstanding ye give them not those things which are needful to the body; what doth it profit? Even so faith, if it hath not works, is dead, being alone. Yea, a man may say, Thou hast faith, and I have works: shew me thy faith without thy works, and I will shew thee my faith by my works. Thou believes that there is one God; thou doest well: the devils also believe, and tremble. But wilt thou know, O vain man, that faith without works is dead? James 2:14-18

And why call ye me, Lord, Lord, and do not the things which I say? Luke 6:46

For another example, Jesus instructs us how to fast. We are to fast in secret and not to boast about it. This teaching also applies to tithing and prayer.

Moreover when ye fast, be not, as the hypocrites, of a sad countenance: for they disfigure their faces, that they may appear unto men to fast. Verily I say unto you, They have their reward. That thou appear not unto men to fast, but unto thy Father which is in secret: and thy Father, which seeth in secret, shall reward thee openly. Matthew 6:16,18

That thine alms may be in secret: and thy Father which seeth in secret himself shall reward thee openly. Matthew 6:4

But thou, when thou prayest, enter into thy closet, and when thou hast shut thy door, pray to thy Father which is in secret; and thy Father which seeth in secret shall reward thee openly. Matthew 6:6

In Isaiah, God was angry with the hypocritical religious activity of their fasting and ignored them and their requests. He told them they should be serving Him by taking care of the hungry and the poor, etc. before He will pour out His blessings upon them:

Wherefore have we fasted, say they, and thou seest not? Wherefore have we afflicted our soul, and thou takest no knowledge? Behold, in the day of your fast ye find your own pleasure, and exact all your labors. Isaiah 58:3 (ASV)

Scripture tells us to love our neighbor as ourselves. *A new commandment I give unto you, That ye love one another; as I have loved you, that ye also love one another* (John 13:34). How do you treat the people around you? We are supposed to always put other people's needs above our own.

- When someone wrongs you, do you turn the other cheek or start thinking of ways to get even?

- When someone hurts you, do you harbor the hurt and pain or do you forgive that person and move on?

- When meeting someone, do you simply accept them or base your acceptance upon how they look, what they do for a living, how much money they make, what they are wearing and what kind of car they drive?

- When looking for a parking spot, do you take the one closest to the building or leave that for someone who may have difficulty walking through the parking lot?

- When shoveling or snowblowing your sidewalk, do you stop before you get to your neighbor's or do you do theirs too?

- When going to the hospital or nursing home to see a relative or friend, do you ever stop in on someone else who may not have had visitors for days – or weeks?

- When cooking or baking, do you make a little extra to take to share at the office, at church or with a lonely neighbor?

- Do you have a servant's heart – putting all others above yourself, or are you too busy with your own concerns?

There are so many things we could be doing that really wouldn't take much extra time or effort, yet they would really make someone else's day.

I remember when I was growing up, my mother would send me over to the neighbor's house to practice my piano lesson. This woman was about four feet tall, about 80 lbs and about 80 some years old – which to me was very old. She had been recently widowed and I am sure, very lonely. She lived in this very large, scary, very dark, old house. Everything in it seemed so ancient. I am sure she had newspapers and magazines that were 30 or 40 years old. She would always try to give me store-bought packaged cookies that must have been at least 10 years old. The point of the story is, I had to practice 30 minutes a day, regardless, and if I did it at the neighbor's house it would give her a lot of joy just to have the company.

If you walk the dog, why not ask a friend to go with. They may not have a dog, but maybe could use the exercise (and the companionship).

How do you treat your wife? *Likewise, ye husbands, dwell with them according to knowledge, giving honour unto the wife, as unto the weaker vessel, and as being heirs together of the grace of life; that your prayers be not hindered.* 1Peter 3:7

You may need to read that verse twice. It says that husbands should honor the wife (as the weaker vessel), or God may not answer your prayers! Why should God bless us if we are not treating others as we ought to?

3. God may also withhold healing because He wants to bring you into obedience.

We have to totally, completely and perfectly submit to God. We must turn everything in our lives over to Him and let Him have control:

Margee wrote:

I suffered severe pain in my back and leg following an injury the winter of 1988. I was hospitalized for a week. The neurosurgeon's comments to me were, "according to the MRI's you shouldn't be in this much pain. You have two herniated discs but I don't want to operate. I'm not sure that the pain is real to the degree you're experiencing it." When

I asked him if he thought the pain was all in my head, he didn't answer me. I went to physical therapy three times a day and lived on pain killers (Vicadin). After three months, the pain subsided and I resumed my normal life. In 1989 the pain returned, lasting for another three months.

The pain reoccurred in 1991, '93, '95 and in '97. All the while I saw a number of doctors, went through numerous tests and went to therapy - to no benefit or consolation. In '97, a rheumatologist, after ruling out Lupus told me I had fibromyalgia. I said, "You mean you're not going to tell me it's all in my head?" He told me it was a very real disorder and that he could help me. I cried right there in his office, He apologized for the other physicians who had discounted my symptoms because they didn't believe me. This particular flare-up of excruciating pain, swollen lymph nodes and painful swollen joint throughout my entire body lasted six months. There were days I couldn't walk as the pain was so unbearable. I was exhausted and I couldn't sleep, averaging only 3 - 4 hours a night.

The most painful part of the experience was because the doctors would not acknowledge that I was in incredible pain, neither did my husband. When I told him what I had and that it was real, he cried and apologized for not believing me. As he is *not one for crying, this was very meaningful to me.*

The helplessness and depression I felt during my flare-ups is unexplainable. I know my Lord brought me through each episode. He was the only one who understood exactly what I was going through. He knew the smile was masking the pain. I began to close myself off from everyone, the mis-understanding and judgment from others hurt as much as the physical pain.

The fall of 1998 I started going to a Bible study which would greatly affect my life. The women the Lord had waiting for me at that study were and are such a blessing to me. Two of the women I devel-oped a friendship with wanted to continue a Bible study in the summer when the other one ended. We studied the book of James and what a study it was! The friendships formed in that small group that summer are for life. Although, over the next several months, one (the author of this book) moved out of state, and the youngest of us, who had been bat-tling anorexia/bulimia, died. She was the same age as my oldest daughter, just 23.

I was alone with Michelle when she died. It was 4-16-00, Palm Sunday. After church I told my hus-band that I needed to spend some time with Michelle at the hospital where she had been for sev-eral days. I went in to her hospital room and her parents stepped out. I read Psalms 139 to her. She folded her hands, closed her eyes and listened. She asked what our pastor spoke on that day. It was on Acts 1:1-10. Shortly after reading the scripture (on the ascension of Christ) to her, Michelle, joined our Savior.

Afterwards, I realized that soon after I stopped praying for her healing and started prayed for her peace and for God's mercy as she was in such incredible pain, that God took her home.

Two days later I attended the weekly prayer meeting at our church. I had never gone before and wanted to be supportive of our church. I was not thinking about myself and I did not ask for prayer of any sort for myself. Because of that, they did not pray for me.

That night I went to bed and was awoken by an electrical humming sound and the feeling of an electrical current that started in my toes and moved up my body. I couldn't open my eyes. I couldn't move. I could feel an incredible energy slowly moving through my whole body and I knew I was being healed. It was like every part of my body was being held in God's hands. The room was aglow – I could see the red through my closed eyelids – and I could feel an incredible warmth.

Since then, I have not had a flare-up when one would otherwise would have arisen and I know that I am Fibromyalgia free. I give my Lord all the glory and praise. The Lord has shown me so many things since that time. He showed me how unforgiving I had been to individuals in my life who had hurt me or my loved ones.

God was saying, "Look what I did for you! I healed you!" He showed me He had forgiven me, but I was not forgiving myself. He showed me how I was carrying a burden of sorrow, which would turn to a hideous anger, rage and then vengeance. He showed me when I did this is when my flare-ups would occur. "Wherefore, my beloved brethren, let every man be swift to hear, slow to speak, slow to wrath." James 1:19

He showed me how many people I was harboring resentments towards who I needed to forgive – all of them. I saw how I just needed to let Him love me through the trials, knowing that God is in control and that things happen in His perfect timing – not ours. God's way is the only right way.

"My brethren, count it all joy when ye fall into divers temptations; Knowing this, that the trying of your faith worketh patience." James 1:2-3

What I was healed from was not from fibromyalgia, I was healed and relieved from the burden of my attempts to control situations that are not in my control. I need to turn over all my trials and sorrows to God and leave them there with Him.

He also showed me how before my healing when I was spending time with Michelle that it was one of the rare occasions when I had my eyes completely off of myself. I had all my trust on the Lord. I had forgotten to eat and prayed like I've never prayed before. I know His Spirit lives inside of us. 1 John 2:24 says, "Therefore let that abide in you which you heard form the beginning. If what you heard from the beginning abides in you, you also will abide in the Son and in the Father."

I know He wants us to love others (including whose who have hurt us), to think of and pray for others rather than constantly focusing on ourselves and our circumstances.

In John 13:34, Jesus said, "A new commandment I give to you, that you love one another; as I have loved you, that you also love one another." Also, in 1 John 4:7-10, "Beloved, let us love one another, for love is of God; and everyone who loves is born of God and knows God. He who does not love does not know God, for God is love. In this the love of God was manifested toward us, that God has sent His only begotten Son into the world, that we might live through Him. In this is love, not that we loved God, but that He first loved us and sent His Son to be the propitiation for our sins. Beloved, if God so loved us, we also ought to love one another. I know that our Lord pours out His mercy upon us daily. We need to recognize that our lives here on earth are short and God gives us numerous occasions to share His love with others. I hope this encourages you to be bold and loving, in His Spirit. Psalm 103:1-3 says, Bless the Lord, O my soul; And all that is within me, bless His holy name! Bless the Lord, O my soul, and forget not all His benefits: Who forgives all your iniquities, Who heals all your diseases.

4. Are you harboring feelings of doubt, guilt, or unworthiness?

Satan can really beat us up if we let him. We may feel all sorts of things making us feel unworthy of God's full blessings. It is important to realize the difference between conviction and condemnation. Conviction is from God. It leads to repentance and brings us closer to God. Condemnation is from Satan, the liar. It pulls us away from our relationship from God as we feel guilty for past sin in our life. If we have repented from those sins and asked for forgiveness, there is no reason to feel guilty any longer.

There is therefore now no condemnation to them which are in Christ Jesus, who walk not after the flesh, but after the Spirit. Romans 8:1

5. Where are your priorities?

No man can serve two masters: for either he will hate the one, and love the other; or else he will hold to the one, and despise the other. Ye cannot serve God and mammon. Matthew 6:24

For where your treasure is, there will your heart be also. Luke 12:34

Are you willing to give up anything for Christ? Are you willing to do whatever it takes to please God? Are you willing to do whatever it is that God asks?

What if that means spending less time with your family? What if that means not getting married and not having a family of your own? What if that means

83

changing jobs or moving to a new area? Obedience to God is required before He will bless us.

And a certain ruler asked Him, saying, Good Master, what shall I do to inherit eternal life? And Jesus said unto him, Why callest thou me good? None is good, save one, that is, God. Thou knowest the commandments, Do not commit adultery, Do not kill, Do not steal, Do not bear false witness, Honour thy father and thy mother. And he said, All these have I kept from my youth up. Now when Jesus heard these things, He said unto him, Yet lackest thou one thing: sell all that thou hast, and distribute unto the poor, and thou shalt have treasure in heaven: and come, follow me. And when he heard this, he was very sorrowful: for he was very rich. And when Jesus saw that he was very sorrowful, He said, How hardly shall they that have riches enter into the kingdom of God! For it is easier for a camel to go through a needle's eye, than for a rich man to enter into the kingdom of God. Luke 18:18-25

6. His ways are not our ways

Remember, we just don't always understand the ways of God and His purposes for the circumstances of our lives. And, because He is God, and we are not, as He reminded Job, we are not even to question Him.

When discussing healing, people will often refer to individuals who became ill, prayed for themselves and received prayer for healing, but were not healed – or died. Or they will talk about someone who died suddenly, without warning, early in life. Death is often viewed as "a let down" or "a negative thing."

As a Christian, death is something we should look forward to. Why would we want to be here on earth in pain and suffering in our broken down, sinful decrepid bodies, when we could be in heaven with the Father in our new perfect bodies? This is the ultimate healing.

We are confident, I say, and willing rather to be absent from the body, and to be present with the Lord. 2 Corinthians 5:8

It is natural to mourn the loss of a loved one and it is only normal that we would miss them, but if they were a believer, we should rejoice in the fact that they are now with the Father.

Death is Not Losing – Death Brings A New Glorious Body

There is nothing wrong with the Christian longing to have a perfect, resurrected body.

For we that are in [this] tabernacle do groan, being burdened: not for that we would be unclothed, but clothed upon, that mortality might be swallowed up of life. 2 Chronicles 5:4

Paul compares our bodies to tents – flimsy, temporary structures. Our bodies are frail, vulnerable, wasting away and do not represent the whole person. There is much more to us than our physical bodies.

(Just as we are to love one another for who we are, not for what we do – because we all fall short – we all sin).

Our future bodies will be specially designed by God to suit the permanent environment of eternity and heaven. The body of flesh is a heavy burden, susceptible to aches, pains and various other discomforts – the stress and calamities of life are a heavy load. But believers also groan because of the burden of a body of sin, and the many corruptions that are still remaining and raging in them. It is a constant struggle. We complain, *O wretched man that I am*! (Romans 7:24).

Instead of looking forward to relief from this burden, many people fear and dread death. I question what could there possibly be on earth that is worth holding onto? If there *is* something, this is separating you from the Father. If this is true for you, you should closely examine your relationship with God. If your relationship is secure with God, there is no reason that you should not desire to be with Him in the total peace and happiness of another life, in our permanent heavenly home.

Matthew Henry writes that all Christians should earnestly desire to be clothed in blessed immortality in heaven. Consider death as merely a separation of soul and body, not to be dreaded, but rather desired and considered a passage to glory. The true believer is willing to die rather than live, to be absent from the body, that we may be present with the Lord – to put off these rags of mortality that we may put on the robes of glory!

Death will strip us of the clothing of flesh and put an end to all our troubles here below. In heaven there will be no sickness, no physical discomfort, no mourning and no sorrow. All our needs will be perfectly met.

They shall be delivered out of all their troubles, and shall have washed their robes and made them white in the blood of the Lamb. Revelation 7:14

For our conversation is in heaven; from whence also we look for the Saviour, the Lord Jesus Christ: Who shall change our vile body, that it may be fashioned like unto His glorious body, according to the working whereby He is able even to subdue all things unto himself. Phillipians 3:20-21

I am not saying that death is an easy thing to deal with. But when someone is close to death, especially when there is great physical pain and suffering, the encouragement that we will receive new and perfect bodies can be a great comfort.

Sharon's cancer had spread into her bones – first her clavicle, then her hip and spine. The cancer demolished her frail body creating great pain until she died. She essentially became a quadriplegic, totally relying on her family and friends to care for all her needs. She had just turned 42 years of age and had three children, ages 9, 12 and 14. At that time, in the early '80s, there was no such thing as hospice, so my mother and others would go over to help out and pray with her. Sharon had a tremendous faith and I imagine the situation was much harder on her husband, family and people around her than for Sharon herself. It is hard to understand the ways of God. Sometimes we are just not meant to.

In another individual dying of bone cancer (which is very painful for those of you unfamiliar with this type of cancer), God was able to use her in this situation to His glory. Howard wrote:

When my mother was dying of cancer of the bone, I had not been to church in over 30 years. My mother a very loving, friendly person, well liked by everyone and seeing her in such great pain really brought up the question of "Why?" At the same time, I strongly sensed a calling to "come home." It was so profound that I told my wife I wanted to go to a local church I had heard about. This was truly a great time of revelation for me – the shepherd will leave his flock to search out one lost sheep.

Note: The cover drawing for this book was done by Howard.

We can be comforted by the fact that God is in control. He does have a perfect plan, regardless of whether or not it is ever revealed to us. Great pain, chronic pain, a critical health problem or a diagnosis of a terminal illness, indicating that death is near, can be a tremendous burden if we try to carry it ourselves. The Bible instructs us to give our burdens to Christ and to draw strength from spending quiet time with Him. *For thus saith the Lord GOD, the Holy One of Israel; In returning and rest shall ye be saved; in quietness and in confidence shall be your strength: and ye would not.* Isaiah 30:15

Attitude and Health

The way we think has a direct impact on our health. If we complain, have stress, anxiety, worry, doubt, depression, anger and other negative emotions, they all have detrimental effects on our health. We have difficulty sleeping, our eating habits change, we either lose our appetite or we may suddenly start eating everything in sight. Our blood pressure goes up, our immune system weakens, we become more susceptible to colds and flu, we get cold sores, our allergies or arthritis acts up, we can even begin losing our hair or find it turning gray. It's a fact. Under stress, the rate at which we use protein, B Vitamins, zinc and other important nutrients increases. If they are not replenished to accommodate for the loss, something is eventually going to suffer. Because our hair is not considered "vital" by the body (like the blood, brain or heart), it is one of the things that suffers first. The body is designed to protect the vital organs. Eventually, however, any tissue or organ in the body can experience the impact of stress and other negative emotions.

God does not want us to worry, He wants us to rely

upon Him for all our needs. Matthew wrote about the needlessness of worry, anxiety and stress.

> *Therefore I say unto you, Take no thought for your life, what ye shall eat, or what ye shall drink; nor yet for your body, what ye shall put on. Is not the life more than meat, and the body than raiment? Behold the fowls of the air: for they sow not, neither do they reap, nor gather into barns; yet your heavenly Father feedeth them. Are ye not much better than they?* Matthew 6:25-26

> *But seek ye first the kingdom of God, and his righteousness; and all these things shall be added unto you.* Matthew 6:33

When we allow ourselves to become stressed, anxious, angry, envious or to experience other negative emotions, we are focusing on ourselves and our circumstances rather than on God. As soon as we take our focus off of Him, we lose our peace.

Depression and feeling sorry for ourselves are very common for those who have a chronic health problem—especially those in chronic pain. It is so prevalent that depression is often listed as a symptom of health problems such as chronic fatigue, arthritis or fibromyalgia.

A cheerful look brings joy to the heart, and good news gives health to the bones.

Proverbs 15:30

Denise wrote:

> *I was raised in a Christian home, but was not attending church and was pretty much living my life my way. I was experiencing migraine headaches which made it difficult to work and my finances started to suffer as well. It was hard to not be depressed. I went to one doctor after another and no one could tell me what was wrong with me. They put me on one medication after another, but nothing helped. I just got more depressed. I sat around feeling sorry for myself. Some of my old bad habits even started creeping back into my life, which just made me more depressed. God was definitely trying to tell me something!*

Sound familiar? This type of experience is actually quite common, especially among women. We all like to have our pity parties. We all feel sorry for ourselves and ask God why this had to happen to us. Chronic pain is no cake walk. I too suffered from headaches – which were aggravated by stress. The publishing business is centered on deadlines and the bottom line is deadlines can be stressful – ask any accountant during tax season, any college student during finals, any emergency room personnel, any member of the police department– the list could go on and on. Stress is a part of life in this world and the key is to not let stress rule you.

You cannot let pain rule your life either. This is exactly what Satan wants. Satan loves to see you wallowing in self pity and feelings of desperation. How can you serve God if you are all caught up in yourself and your pain? To survive, you must turn the pain over to God every day. Every single day.

Depression often includes isolating yourself or giving up. It can make you withdraw from life – from doing the things that you previously found enjoyment and satisfaction in, such as spending time or talking with friends and family, being involved in church and community activities, working, and doing crafts or hobby activities. Dropping out just makes you more depressed. This is exactly what Satan wants.

The Sin of Depression

If we are depressed, where is our focus? On ourselves. This form of selfishness, and self pity, is counter productive.

And not only so, but we glory in tribulations also: knowing that tribulation worketh patience; And patience, experience; and experience, hope: And hope maketh not ashamed; because the love of God is shed abroad in our hearts by the Holy Ghost which is given unto us. For when we were yet without strength, in due time, Christ died for the ungodly. Romans 5:3-6

Take glory in our tribulations? That's not so easy to do if we are looking at our suffering from our own perspective. God tells us to look at it from His perspective, and He tells us that He will use each trial for His glory. While in the midst of our heartache or physical pain, we may not understand why this is happening to us, why it has to be so hard, why it has to hurt so much, and it is possible that we never will understand. It is our human nature to want answers. If you search the scriptures and pray, God may tell you, "Trust Him, He knows what He is doing."

King David sought the comfort of God in his many trials. The Psalms are a wonderful place to "hang out" for those who are truly hurting. David was no different from us. He loved God. He sinned. God punished Him. He suffered and complained. He humbled himself, repented and cried out to God for forgiveness. God forgave him, just like He forgives us. It is a great example for us.

Have mercy upon me, O LORD, for I am in trouble: mine eye is consumed with grief, yea, my soul and my belly. For my life is spent with grief, and my years with sighing: my strength faileth because of mine iniquity, and my bones are consumed. I was a reproach among all mine enemies, but especially among my neighbors, and a fear to mine acquaintance: they that did see me without fled from me. I am forgotten as a dead man out of mind: I am like a broken vessel. For I have heard the slander of many: fear was on every side: while they took counsel together against me, they devised to take away my life. But I trusted in thee, O LORD: I said, Thou art my God. Psalms 31:9-14

O LORD, rebuke me not in thy wrath: neither chasten me in thy hot displeasure. For thine arrows stick fast in me, and thy hand presseth me sore. There is no soundness in my flesh because of thine anger; neither is there any rest in my bones because of my sin. For mine iniquities are gone over mine head: as an heavy burden they are too heavy for me. My wounds stink and are corrupt because of my foolishness. I am troubled; I am bowed down greatly; I go mourning all the day long. For my loins are filled with a loathsome disease: and there is no soundness in my flesh. I am feeble and sore broken: I have roared by reason of the disquietness of my heart. Lord, all my desire is before thee; and my groaning is not hid from thee. My heart panteth, my strength faileth me: as for the light of mine eyes, it also is gone from me. My lovers and my friends stand aloof from my sore; and my kinsmen stand afar off. They also that seek after my life lay snares for me: and they that seek my hurt speak mischievous things, and imagine deceits all the day long. But I, as a deaf man, heard not; and I was as a dumb man that openeth not his mouth. Thus, I was as a man that heareth not, and in whose mouth are no reproofs. For in thee, O LORD, do I hope: thou wilt hear, O Lord my God. For I said, Hear me, lest otherwise they should rejoice over me: when my foot slippeth, they magnify themselves against me. For I am ready to halt, and my sorrow is continually before me. For I will declare mine iniquity; I will be sorry for my sin. But mine enemies are lively, and they are strong: and they that hate me wrongfully are multiplied. They also that render evil for good are mine adversaries; because I follow the thing that good is. Forsake me not, O LORD: O my God, be not far from me. Psalms 38:1-21

Blessed is that man that maketh <u>the LORD</u> his trust. Psalms 40:4

Does it say 'blessed is that man that maketh *alcohol* his trust?'

or antidepressants?

or pain killers?

or sleeping pills?

or food?

or Alanon?

or Alcoholics Anonymous?

or making money?

or buying toys?

or sex?

or your spouse?

or your psychiatrist?

or your friends?

These are some of the things that we are turning to *instead* of God. None of these things will truly give you the lasting comfort and true peace you are seeking.

They have heard that I sigh: there is none to comfort me: all mine enemies have heard of my trouble; they are glad that thou hast done it: thou wilt bring the day that thou hast called, and they shall be like unto me. Lamentations 1:21

*For the idols have spoken vanity, and the divin-
ers have seen a lie, and have told false dreams;
they comfort in vain: therefore they went their way
as a flock, they were troubled, because there was
no shepherd.* Zechariah 10:2

If we turn to anything other than God in our times
of stress, depression, anxiousness, etc. it becomes like
a false god – an idol. Does a pan of brownies or a bag
of donuts make you feel any better? No, it makes you
feel worse and if you keep doing it, you are likely to
make God angry (and overweight as well).

We need to go to God – and to His word to get the
only lasting, meaningful, sincere comfort:

*Remember the word unto thy servant, upon
which thou hast caused me to hope. This is my comfort in my affliction: for thy word hath quickened me.*
Psalm 119: 49-50

*For whatsoever things were written aforetime
were written for our learning, that we through
patience and comfort of the scriptures might have
hope.* Romans 15:4

*O Lord my God, in thee do I put my trust: save
me from all them that persecute me, and deliver me.*
Psalm 7:1

*Beloved, think it not strange concerning the
fiery trial which is to try you, as though some
strange thing happened unto you: But rejoice, inas-*

*much as ye are partakers of Christ's sufferings;
that, when His glory shall be revealed, ye may be
glad also with exceeding joy.* 1 Peter 4:12-13

This is such a great scripture, because this is just how we are. In our humanness, we feel sorry for ourselves as though no one else on earth has ever had to deal with what we are going through.

Depression and emotional trauma play a significant role in the ability of our immune system to function optimally. The immune system is controlled by various hormones in the blood stream and by neurochemicals and nerves. Negative emotions such as depression, grief, anger, bitterness, hatred, etc., are known to increase the production of certain hormones which suppress the activity of the immune system.

One of the most common precursors of cancer is a traumatic loss (death of loved one, loss of job, etc.) or feeling of emptiness in one's life (divorce or children have all left home). Emotional loss that is not properly dealt with hampers the body's immune response which would otherwise keep potentially cancerous cells (which are present in the body at all times) under check.

In *Love, Medicine & Miracles*, Bernie Siegal, M.D. wrote, *"The simple truth is, happy people generally don't get sick. One's attitude toward oneself is the single most important factor in healing or staying well. Those who are at peace with themselves and their immediate surroundings have far fewer serious illnesses than those who do not."*

The Sin of Stress

Henry Blackaby and Claude King make an excellent statement in their book, *Experiencing God.* They state, "What I believe about God will determine what I do and how I live." Are you putting your trust in God, or are you stressing out, living your life in anxiety and fear?

Do you realize that worry and allowing yourself to become stressed over your circumstances is sinful? By worrying excessively and wasting mental energy trying to figure something out that you have no control over, you are telling God that you do not trust Him and His ability to handle things in the way that He sees fit?

The Body Hates Stress (and negativity)

Stress is a negative emotion with no positive effects whatsoever. When stress starts to build, your body fights back. First, it releases stress hormones, such as cortisol, epinephrine and norepinephrine, which make your heart rate rise, your metabolism speed up, your muscles tense, and your breathing become faster and more shallow.

These reactions stem from the fight-or-flight response – the body's involuntary, split-second reaction to danger. Since the body can't tell the difference

---

A sound heart is the life of the flesh: but envy the rottenness of the bones.

Proverbs 14:30

between a physical threat and a mental one, it can sound the fight-or-flight alarm dozens of times a day, regardless of whether the reaction is caused by your boss's yelling or a semi-truck bearing down on you on the freeway. Your body can go into a chronic state of vigilance. Ultimately, all the ongoing everyday signals can damage your heart, blood vessels and brain.

Stress affects your appetite and your eating habits, causing you to lose or gain weight: *Fools, because of their transgression, and because of their iniquities, are afflicted. Their soul abhorreth all manner of meat; and they draw near unto the gates of death* (Psalms107:17-18).

Stress affects your sleep, your concentration and memory. Stress is physically draining and will make you feel exhausted. Whatever inherent weakness you may have will surface – nervous habits, arthritis, headaches, allergies, skin problems, etc. The body cannot function properly for very long in this "flight or fight" mode, and eventually, it will begin to suffer.

"Stress accelerates the onset of age-related diseases," says Allen J. Elkin, Ph.D., director of the Stress Management and Counseling Center in New York City. "There's virtually no part of the body that escapes the ravages of stress."

When you are stressed-out, your body produces more free radicals, which are naturally-occurring unstable oxygen molecules in the body that attack and damage cells. Free radicals speed up the aging process and create all sorts of health problems. "Free radicals are responsible for most signs of aging, including cataracts, macular degeneration, circulatory problems,

Health Problems associated with stress, bitterness, hostility, animosity, hatred, anxiety, fear and other negative emotions:

Addictions (and nervous habits such as nail biting, over-eating, drinking, smoking, etc.)

Premature Aging

Allergies

Asthma

Cancer

Chronic Fatigue

Fibromyalgia

Depression

Digestive Disorders (Irritable bowel, etc.)

Hair Loss

Heart Palpitations/Irregular heart beat

Heart Disease

High Blood Pressure

Hives

Depressed Immunity (Increases susceptibility to colds, flu, cold sores, allergies and all other health problems)

Memory Loss/Loss of Concentration

Migraine Headaches

Mood Swings/Irritability

Panic/Anxiety Disorders

Sleep Disorders

Weight Problems (loss or gain) **and Obesity**

gray hair, dry skin and wrinkles, and even some cancers," says Paul J. Rosch, M.D., clinical professor of medicine and psychiatry at New York Medical College in Valhalla and president of the American Institute of Stress in Yonkers, New York.

Many physical problems can begin with the poison of negativity – anxiety, bitterness, hostility, animosity, hatred, etc. When we get upset, tensed and stressed, the heart rate and blood pressure increase and the body produces and releases hormones such as cortisol. In high levels, cortisol interferes with our ability to sleep (inhibits our REM "deep" sleep), disrupts concentration, interferes with the body's ability to regulate inflammation and production and proper functioning of other hormones (such as progesterone) and has many other negative effects. These all have detrimental effects on the immune system. High blood pressure is one of the risk factors for heart disease.

By allowing ourselves to become stressed out by our circumstances, we are telling God that we don't trust Him and that our circumstances are more important than He is, because that is where all our attention is. We will be a lot healthier if we walk in obedience to God.

Marcia wrote:
My health problems began in 1971 when I was 25 years old and pregnant with my second child. I developed severe nerve pain sending sharp shooting pains throughout my body and head. After seeing several specialists over a five-year period, I was diagnosed with M.S. at the University of Minnesota

and the Mayo Clinic. I went through two years of severe depression. We then had three children under the age of seven.

In 1977, my husband was diagnosed with a malignant brain tumor. This was a spiritual awakening for both of us. I had spent two years crying out to God for myself and for my healing. We were now both terrified. We joined a charismatic Catholic prayer group that met weekly. We did not miss a week for the next five years and came to lean fully on God My husband died six years after his diagnosis in 1983 in perfect peace.

Stress has been a huge part of my life and I am sure it contributed to my health problems.

In 1986, doctors claimed that my M.S. was definite. I attended M.S. meetings and desperately searched for a cure, each day living in pain.

Then in 1996, another doctor claimed I had no evidence of M.S. whatsoever and claimed that all those years I had been misdiagnosed because they didn't know what was wrong with me. I was relieved that it was not M.S., but angry with the physicians who had given me a wrong diagnosis, just to give me an answer. All the while, my condition was getting worse.

I became extremely depressed and my health problems progressed to the point where I was even suicidal. My nerve pain had increased and I had developed joint pain and other symptoms as well. It was so uncomfortable that I had to stop working. My doctor prescribed antidepressants and diagnosed *fibromyalgia, as I had most of it's symptoms.*

At age 54, I now realize while it is impossible to live stress-free in this world, one must not focus on it. The one and only thing that keeps me going is my faith in God and I feel His presence at all times in my life. I would not trade my experiences as they have brought me closer to Him.

The loss of my Mother to cancer at age 11 and my best friend and husband when I was 36, showed me that the only one I can count on is God.

Come unto Me, all ye that labor and are heavy laden, and I will give you rest. Take My yoke upon you, and learn of Me; for I am meek and lowly in heart: and ye shall find rest unto your souls. For My yoke is easy, and My burden is light. Matthew 11:28-30

Once you start winning the stress battle, it's almost a sure thing that you will stay healthier. The opposite of stress is peace. The emotion of true peace is proven in clinical trials to enhance health, and speed healing and recovery.

Peace and health are what God wants for us. The only way to obtain true peace is to put your total trust in Him. Take your focus off of yourself and your circumstances and put it onto Him and what He can do for you. Nothing else is going to fill that void that we are all looking for in our life. Material things, money, even family and loved ones simply can never provide the peace that passes all understanding that we can **only** get from Him.

God wants us to give our burdens to Him. As long as you continue to try to fight the battle (without Christ), you will not have peace. You can't have peace, because you can never win. The battles you are trying to fight are of a spiritual nature.

For we wrestle not against flesh and blood, but against principalities, against powers, against the rulers of the darkness of this world, against spiritual wickedness in high places. Ephesians 6:12

If you believe that God will do what He promises, the Holy Spirit can restore your confidence to realize that God is in control – He has already won the battle and you can have peace.

This has to be done every day. In certain circumstances, you may need to go to Him and give your burdens to Him several times a day. There is nothing wrong with that, this is not a sign of weakness. It is actually a sign of strength and confidence in God. I have had days when circumstances were such that I felt the need to spend most of the day with the Lord and in the Word. I felt like I needed to repeat over and over, "God is in control. God is in control."

I can do all things through Christ which strengtheneth me. Phillipians 4:13

Peace gives us confidence in our ability to face our circumstances, no matter how challenging they are. This is a very important aspect of obtaining and maintaining what God wants for us. The author of the letter to the Hebrews tells us not to throw away our confidence. *Cast not away therefore your confidence, which hath great recompence of reward. For ye have need of patience, that, after ye have done the will of God, ye might receive the promise.* Hebrews 10:35-36

Be of good courage, and he shall strengthen your heart, all ye that hope in the LORD. Psalms 31:24

The Power of Belief

Each of the following stories tell how individuals who believed that they could be healed, were. In Acts, the writer (Luke) tells the story of how a crippled man was instantly healed after Peter instructed him to walk.

And a certain man lame from his mother's womb was carried, whom they laid daily at the gate of the temple which is called Beautiful, to ask alms of them that entered into the temple; Who seeing Peter and John about to go into the temple asked for alms. And Peter, fastening his eyes upon him with John, said, "Look on us." And he gave heed unto them, expecting to receive something of them. Then Peter said, "Silver and gold have I none; but such as I have give I thee: In the name of Jesus Christ of Nazareth rise up and walk." And he took him by the right hand, and lifted him up: and immediately his feet and ankle bones received strength. And he leaping up stood, and walked, and entered with them into the temple, walking, and leaping, and praising God. Acts 3:2-8

When Jesus was traveling from Judea into Galilee he met a nobleman, whose son was sick at Capernaum.

When he heard that Jesus was come out of Judea into Galilee, he went unto him, and besought him that he would come down, and heal his son; for he was at the point of death. Jesus therefore said unto him, Except ye see signs and wonders, ye will in no wise believe. The nobleman saith unto him, Sir, come down ere my child die. Jesus saith unto him, Go thy way; thy son liveth. The man believed the word that Jesus spake unto him, and he went his way. And as he was now going down, his servants met him, saying, that his son lived. So he inquired of them the hour when he began to amend. They said therefore unto him, Yesterday at the seventh hour the fever left him. So the father knew that it was at that hour in which Jesus said unto him, Thy son liveth: and himself believed, and his whole house. John 4:47-54

And, behold, there came a leper and worshiped him, saying, Lord, if thou wilt, thou canst make me clean. And Jesus put forth his hand, and touched him, saying, I will; be thou clean. And immediately his leprosy was cleansed. Matthew 8:2-3

Muriel wrote:

Alma had a daughter, Susan, born with one leg shorter than the other. The doctor decided since she was so little they would wait a couple months before attempting any corrective surgery on her. Every day

Alma prayed for those legs of her baby to be of equal length. She went back to the doctor at the appointed time, he measured the legs and they were perfectly equal. He asked her what she had done and she said, "I just prayed for her." This changed her life. She realized God was real and He really heard a "mother's heart" and that He loved everybody – big or small, that all of her prayers were heard by Him, and that prayer changes things.

Alma has had many miracles in her life but the most recent is a healing from shingles. She had it in the "bottom" area and it was so bad and painful she could not even sit down. She had this condition for about seven days and had been praying continually for her healing. One day, while laying on the couch, she felt an immense heat run through her bottom. She immediately sat up. The pain was gone and all the lesions dried up in the next few days. She realized that she had been completely dependent upon God and He had been so good to heal her. Prayer really works. You just have to cry out to Him – He does hear and answer you. Isaiah 58:9 says, Then shalt thou call, and the LORD shall answer; thou shalt cry, and He shall say, Here I am.

If my people, which are called by my name, shall humble themselves, and pray, and seek my face, and turn from their wicked ways; then will I hear from heaven, and will forgive their sin, and will heal their land. 2 Chronicles 7:14

The Power of Love

Just as stress, anger, hostility, envy and anxiety are negative emotions with negative impacts upon our health, the positive emotions of love and joy have a positive impact on our health. Love has the power to heal us physically, spiritually and emotionally.

If you express sincere Godly love to a person who is sick, it will certainly aid in their recovery. We all want to feel loved. When we are in pain or not feeling well, as we experience the physical frailness of our flesh, the desire to be loved can be even stronger. It is an awful feeling to be sick and be all alone. This is one of the reasons it is so important to visit the sick and the elderly, to show them God's love and aid in their healing. Loving one another is God's commandment.

This is my commandment, That ye love one another, as I have loved you. John 15:12

Darlene wrote:

He came up from the ER in the early afternoon. From the report called to me by the ER nurse, I knew I was in for it. He was experiencing food poisoning and for the last few days had been vomiting. By the time he arrived on the unit, it hadn't magically stopped. The common antiemetics had not seemed to reduce his misery in the slightest. In his late 60s, he spoke as though he had little education. Granted, he had been sick for awhile, but hygiene was obviously not one of his strong points. He was unkept and a little "rough around the edges." Our communi-

cation was difficult with his southern accent and my northern accent, as well as his partial hearing loss. Honestly, I have never seen someone so sick that was still able to stand up!

For the last few hours of my shift ,I tried all that I could to make him more comfortable, keep his dehydration from getting worse and stop his vomiting, so that he could get some rest. He hadn't slept in days! Doctors came and left orders which I carried out, but nothing seemed to help.

As my shift came to an end, I gave his report to the next nurse and then said a prayer as I knocked on his door. How helpless I felt in trying to make him feel better. Had I done anything to help him at all?

I expressed my regrets to him that I was not able to help him very much. I told him that all I knew to do was to pray and asked him if I do so before I left. He agreed and I took his hand and appealed to the Great Healer who I know is sympathetic to our pain and discomfort. When I finished there were tears in his eyes and I was compelled to hug him despite the smell, etc. In nursing school I was taught that this was not considered "professional." It is never considered professional in the medical field to admit that you really are totally powerless to make the least difference and that you have no idea what to do to make someone better, but I didn't care. I decided at that moment to never let my pride get in the way of pointing my patients to the only One that can truly help them.

Then, the unexpected − no, he was not miraculously better – something even more unexpected! With tears in his eyes, he thanked me and simply said, "I love you." I then did the most "unprofessional" thing of my entire nursing career. With complete honesty, I told him that I loved him too. I was not flattered by his comment or embarrassed. I felt as though I was looking into the eyes of Christ Himself. I could not have felt more loved and valued if he had been the most handsome, young, available man in the world!

I tell this story because it has changed my life. It has adjusted my attitude, and opened my eyes to clearly see myself as I am – prideful, and yet truly helpless to make an impact on others without God. I will never look for association again from only the young, healthy and vibrant. True contentment comes by seeing each one as equal in the sight of God and giving of myself in humble service as though I were serving Jesus Himself! This is possible only by looking past outward appearances and deep into the potential that each one has! The image of God was created into all of us and the reason I don't see it is because I don't look for it!

And the King shall answer and say unto them, Verily I say unto you, In as much as you have done it unto one of the least of these my brethren, you have done it unto me. Matthew 25:40

What is Our Role?

Thou shalt therefore keep the commandments, and the statutes, and the judgments, which I command thee this day, to do them. Wherefore it shall come to pass, if ye hearken to these judgments, and keep, and do them, that the LORD thy God shall keep unto thee the covenant and the mercy which he sware unto thy fathers: And He will love thee, and bless thee, and multiply thee: He will also bless the fruit of thy womb, and the fruit of thy land, thy corn, and thy wine, and thine oil, the increase of thy kine, and the flocks of thy sheep, in the land which He sware unto thy fathers to give thee...

And the LORD will take away from thee all sickness, and will put none of the evil diseases of Egypt, which thou knowest, upon thee; but will lay them upon all them that hate thee. . . The Lord will keep you free from every disease. Deuteronomy 7:11-13, 15

Be not wise in thine own eyes: fear the LORD, and depart from evil. It shall be health to thy navel, and marrow to thy bones. Proverbs 3:7-8

What Are You Doing For God?

As Christians, meaning we have accepted Christ into our heart, as our personal Lord and Savior, we strive to be like Christ. This practice of sanctification is a life-long process which cannot exist without a personal relationship with God. It involves obedience and service.

Let this mind be in you, which was also in Christ Jesus: Who, being in the form of God, thought it not robbery to be equal with God: But made Himself of no reputation, and took upon Him the form of a servant, and was made in the likeness of men: And being found in fashion as a man, He humbled himself, and became obedient unto death, even the death of the cross. Phillipians 2:5-8

Do you ever feel like your prayers are a list of all the things that *you* want? Straighten out this person, comfort that person, heal this person, help me get a new job, tell me what to do about this situation, etc.? How much time do you spend asking God what *He* wants from you? What is it that He wants to show you today? How can you serve *Him*?

Verily, verily, I say unto you, Except a corn of wheat fall into the ground and die, it abideth alone: but if it die, it bringeth forth much fruit. He that loveth his life shall lose it; and he that hateth his life in this world shall keep it unto life eternal. If any man serve Me, let him follow Me; and where I am, there shall also My servant be: if any man serve Me, him will my Father honour. John 12:24-26

Earlier I mentioned that God created us for two reasons, to love us and for us to serve Him. If we claim to be Christians we must be serving our Lord. *Faith without works is dead* (James 2:20). Acknowledging that we are children of God means we are acknowledging that He owns us, He paid the price. We don't own our bodies and our lives. We owe our lives to Him and all He asks of us is that we serve Him.

Are you serving God? Or are you caught up in your secular job, going home to watch TV and relax, going to church on the weekend, only to hurry home to catch a game or go fishing or boating or hang out with your friends and family? There is nothing wrong with hanging out with your family, but how much time are you spending with God?

How much more shall the blood of Christ, who through the eternal Spirit offered himself without spot to God, purge your conscience from dead works to serve the living God? Hebrews 9:14

Many people think that in order to serve God they must be a pastor, a missionary in some third-world country, an elder, or that God will ask something of them that they will just not want to do. This is not what being a servant means. It does mean that we need to simply be available to do whatever it is that God calls us to do. We can serve God by being a good wife, by raising Godly children, by helping to wash communion glasses after church, by leading a Bible study, by bringing food to a family that recently lost a loved one or that is having financial trouble, by visiting shut-ins, by helping out at a "soup kitchen," or even by praying for others.

He has a purpose for all of us. If you do not know how God wants you to serve Him, just ask Him. He will tell you. Just listen.

Having predestinated us unto the adoption of children by Jesus Christ to himself, according to the good pleasure of His will. Ephesians 1:5

The eyes of your understanding being enlightened; that ye may know what is the hope of His calling, and what the riches of the glory of His inheritance in the saints. Ephesians 1:18

Behold, I have refined you, but not as silver; I have tested you in the furnace of affliction. For Mine own sake, even for Mine own sake, I will do this: for how should My name be polluted? And I will not give My glory unto another. Isaiah 48:10-11 (NIV)

Sometimes God has to "refine" us to prepare us to serve Him. We may need humbling. We may need compassion. We may need to grow up a little. We may have scales on our eyes blinding us to His truth. We may be judging others or harboring resentment and unforgiveness without realizing what we are doing.

God knows our hearts and He knows exactly how much "refinement" is needed so we can serve Him according to His will.

Share your food with the hungry and open your houses to the poor traveler who has nowhere to stay. Give clothes to those who have nothing and don't forget the needy members of your own family. If you do this My light will shine on you like the morning sun and your healing will be quickly evident. Isaiah 58:7-8

Dr. Ken Johnson, a colleague of mine and fellow servant of God, emailed me this beautiful story he titled, "Small Things with Great Love!"

The day was Thankful Thursday, our "designated day" of service. It's a weekly tradition that my two little girls and I began years ago. Thursday has become our day to go out in the world and make a positive contribution. On this particular Thursday, we had no idea exactly what we were going to do, but we knew that something would present itself.

Driving along a busy Houston road, praying for guidance in our quest to fulfill our weekly Act of Kindness, the noon hour appropriately triggered hunger pangs in my two little ones.

They wasted no time in letting me know, chanting, "McDonald's, McDonald's, McDonald's," as we drove along. I relented and began searching earnestly for the nearest McDonald's. Suddenly I realized that almost every intersection I passed through was occupied by a panhandler. And then it hit me! If my two little ones were hungry, then all these panhandlers must be hungry, too. Perfect! Our Act of Kindness had presented itself. We were going to buy lunch for the panhandlers.

After finding a McDonald's and ordering two

Happy Meals for my girls, I ordered an additional 15 lunches and we set out to deliver them. It was exhilarating. We would pull alongside a panhandler, make a contribution, and tell him or her that we hoped things got better. Then we'd say, "Oh, by the way...here's lunch." And then we would varoom off to the next intersection.

It was the best way to give. There wasn't enough time for us to introduce ourselves or explain what we were going to do, nor was there time for them to say anything back to us. The Act of Kindness was anonymous and empowering for each of us, and we loved what we saw in the rear view mirror: a surprised and delighted person holding up his lunch bag and just looking at us as we drove off. It was wonderful!

We had come to the end of our "route" and there was a small woman standing there, asking for change. We handed her our final contribution and lunch bag, and then immediately made a U-turn to head back in the opposite direction for home.

Unfortunately, the light caught us again and we were stopped at the same intersection where this little woman stood. I was embarrassed and didn't know quite how to behave. I didn't want her to feel obligated to say or do anything. She made her way to our car, so I put the window down just as she started to speak. "No one has ever done anything like this for me before," she said with amazement. I replied, "Well, I'm glad that we were the first." Feeling uneasy, and wanting to move the conversa-

tion along, I asked, "So, when do you think you'll eat your lunch?"

She just looked at me with her huge, tired brown eyes and said, "Oh honey, I'm not going to eat this lunch." I was confused, but before I could say anything, she continued. "You see, I have a little girl of my own at home and she just loves McDonald's, but I can never buy it for her because I just don't have the money. But you know what... tonight she is going to have McDonald's!" I don't know if the kids noticed the tears in my eyes. So many times I had questioned whether our Acts of Kindness were too small or insignificant to really effect change. Yet in that moment, I recognized the truth of Mother Teresa's words: "We cannot do great things – only small things with great love."

The following story shows the heart of a true servant. After Jesus and the disciples ate, Jesus got up and began to wash the feet of his disciples. This menial task was normally done by the lowest servant of the household, the bonds servant, when guests arrived to cleanse the dirt from their feet after walking around in open sandals. There was no servant available and no one else volunteered. But Jesus, waiting until after the meal to emphasize the act, demonstrated what true selfless service is all about by washing the feet of his followers.

He riseth from supper, and laid aside His garments; and took a towel, and girded Himself. After that He poureth water into a basin, and began to

117

wash the disciples' feet, and to wipe them with the towel wherewith He was girded. Then cometh He to Simon Peter: and Peter saith unto Him, "Lord, does thou wash my feet?" Jesus answered and said unto him, What I do thou knowest not now; but thou shalt know hereafter. Peter saith unto Him, Thou shalt never wash my feet. Jesus answered him, If I wash thee not, thou hast no part with me. Simon Peter saith unto Him, Lord, not my feet only, but also my hands and my head. Jesus said to him, He that is washed need not save to wash his feet, but is clean every whit: and ye are clean, but not all. For He knew who should betray him; therefore said He, Ye are not all clean. So after he had washed their feet, and had taken his garments, and was set down again, he said unto them, Know ye what I have done to you? Ye call me Master and Lord: and ye say well; for so I am. If I then, your Lord and Master, have washed your feet; ye also ought to wash one another's feet. For I have given you an example, that ye should do as I have done to you. Verily, verily, I say unto you, The servant is not greater than his lord; neither he that is sent greater than he that sent him. If ye know these things, happy are ye if ye do them. John 13:4-17

Do you ever feel like you don't need to help out in the kitchen or change a diaper because that's women's work? Or that you don't need to go visit people (yep, perfect strangers) at the nursing home because there might be a good game on TV to watch? Do you feel like you don't need to help put chairs away after church because you want to talk business with a client you saw on the other side of church? Would you get up at 5 or 6 a.m. and spend the whole day to have a rummage sale of all the clothes your kids have out-grown and make $17 rather than donate the clothes to the shelter for the needy?

It's all about putting the needs of others ahead of your own. *Let nothing be done through strife or vainglory; but in lowliness of mind let each esteem others better than themselves* (Phillipians 2:3).

How do you treat other people? Do you have a servant's heart? Do you put your own needs above those of others – including those people you may not even like? Are you critical of others? Even judgmental?

His name was Bill. He had wild hair, wore a T-shirt with holes in it, jeans and no shoes. This was literally his wardrobe for his entire four years of college. Bill was kind of esoteric and very, very bright. He became a Christian while attending college. Across the street from the campus was a well dressed, very conservative church. They wanted to develop a ministry to the students, but were not sure how to go about it.

One day Bill decided to go there. He walked in with no shoes, jeans, his T-shirt and wild hair. The service had already started, so Bill started down the aisle looking for a seat. The church was completely packed; he couldn't find a seat. By now people were really looking a bit uncomfortable. but no-one said anything. Bill got closer and closer to the pulpit and, when he realized there were no seats, he just squatted down right on the carpet. (Although perfectly acceptable behavior at a college fellowship, trust me, this had never happened in this church before!)

By now the people were really uptight, and the tension in the air was thick. About this time, the minister realized that from way in the back of the church, a deacon began slowly making his way toward Bill. Now the deacon was in his 80s, had silver-grey hair, and wore a three-piece suit. He was a godly man, very elegant, very dignified and very courtly. He walked with a cane and, as he started walking toward this boy, everyone was saying to themselves that you couldn't blame him for what he was going to do.

How could you expect a man of his age and of his background to understand some college kid on the floor?

It took a long time for the man to reach the young man. The church was utterly silent except for the clicking of the old man's cane. All eyes focused on him. You couldn't hear anyone breathing. The minister couldn't even preach the sermon until the deacon did what he had to do. And then they saw this elderly man drop his cane on the floor. With great difficulty he lowered himself and sat down next to Bill and worshiped with him so he wouldn't be alone.

Everyone choked up with emotion. When the

minister gained control he said, "What I'm about to preach, you will never remember. What you have just seen, you will never forget. Be careful how you live. You may be the only Bible some people ever read."

Let us pray for ourselves that we may, indeed, be a living Bible, serving God, by serving each other.

Dwight wrote:
My initial memory is of painful experiences as I grew up on the farm. My early pain was of confusion and of many various infections – ear, sinus, bladder, etc. During my teen years I had mononucleosis. In the military I suffered from intense joint and back pain. That is when the pharmaceuticals entered into the "treatment program" in a big way. First it was aspirin, then valium, butylzolodine, and indocin – all of which were prescribed in larger and larger doses and never alleviating the pain. There were periods of prescribed bed rest along with the assistance of back braces and walking canes in order to function at a minimal level.

As the pain intensity increased, there were examinations by various experts from military and veterans facilities, as well as the Mayo Clinic. "Nothing can be done" was always the dreaded prognosis!

By the age of 24, I was dealing with psychiatrists who added antidepressants such as Elavil, Triavil, Cogentin, lithium, etc. to the already long list of drugs. At this time I was not only solidifying from arthritis but I had been diagnosed as manic depressive (bi-polar). "Being content" was something I had never experienced, so at the age of 25 I tried to leave this world by attempting suicide. My second attempt was at the age of 36, for I truly felt there was no other "hell" than the one that I had been experiencing for most of my life.

After the second attempt I became resigned to the fact that I was not going forward in any way – so with this enlightenment, I engaged the doctors and switched to Tegretol and then Prozac. By the age of 39, I was a virtual raving lunatic. My body had run out of all physical substance and manifested (fully recompensed) cancer – the "ultimate socially-acceptable disease."

Stepping back in time, I must say, while all these things were happening to me, I searched vigorously for any solution to my condition.

From the ages of 19 to 36, my focus was entirely on nutrition, environmental influences and relationships. All of these aspects were changed frequently with no positive effects on my condition.

At the age of 36, I received Jesus Christ as my Lord and Savior, but had no personal, interactive relationship with Him. At that point my physical, emotional, and mental state went from very bad to even worse! My physical body did not begin healing until three years later when I completely quit going to all of the doctors and refused all pharmaceuticals. After a healing crises that lasted for six months, I began to earnestly seek herbal and spiritual wisdom and understanding. I had completely reached "the end of myself."

Consequently, the teachers were sent my way – line upon line I was led back to the Lord Jesus Christ and the interactive, personal relationship I hold so dearly today. The Lord blessed me with a helpmate (my bride, Barbara) and together we, as led, have founded "From The Garden Ministries" where we share with others the truths of God's will according to our relationship with Him; and how we are to live in this world with the tools and provisions He has so wisely provided. Our bodies were created to heal themselves and He is teaching the Body of Christ how to "come into order" and walk in the wholeness of His Truth. The key to the door of true healing is "repentance and forgiveness" as we "get our house in order" according to the instructions set forth in His Word, beginning "in the garden"!

I am aware now that had I not suffered these many forms of affliction, I would have a difficult time, at best, having compassion for those who are suffering now.

"Who can have compassion on the ignorant, and on them are out of the way; for that he himself also is compassed with infirmity." Hebrews 5:2

Of Jesus Christ it is written, "Though he were a Son, yet learned he obedience by the things which he suffered." Hebrews 5:8

I am unsure at this time where the limits are in healing; as we are experiencing miraculous healing responses to the process that we have been given to teach and share with others. The Lord has no limits; so we pray that His will be done in each and every case brought into our path.

As I write this, I acknowledge that we also are in the process of continuous change; in order to refine and accelerate the cleansing, rejuvenating, and restoring of the physical, emotional, and spiritual body that is called to walk in complete healing and wholeness by the Lord Jesus Christ.

All the while, "the peace that passes all understanding" is enjoyed here at the Barn House and From The Garden Ministries.

Authors note: From The Garden Ministries is a Christian recovery center (The Barn House) in Albany, Oregon ministering to individuals recovering from physical, emotional and spiritual damage.

What About Doctors?

There is so much power attributed to modern medicine, drugs and doctors that many people now just expect that if they go to the doctor when they get sick, they will be made well. First of all, what does this say about our faith in God if He is not who we seek first for all of our troubles?

But seek ye first the kingdom of God, and His righteousness; and all these things shall be added unto you. Matthew 6:33

Seek the LORD and his strength, seek His face continually. 1 Chronicles 16:11

And (King) Asa in the thirty and ninth year of his reign was diseased in his feet, until his disease was exceeding great: yet in his disease he sought not to the LORD, but to the physicians. And Asa slept with his fathers, and died in the one and fortieth year of his reign. 2 Chronicles 16:11-13

Second, doctors are people just like us. There are good doctors (I could even name a few) and there are horrible doctors. And... all doctors make mistakes.

Third, most drugs do more harm than good. If they did not have side effects, they would not be prescription drugs, and they would be available over the counter. However, over-the-counter medications have side effects too.

One problem I have with modern medicine is that it seems 99% of the time the focus of the treatment is on the symptoms not the cause of the problem. I will never forget going to visit my father in the hospital after his second coronary bypass surgery. I arrived just as he was receiving his evening meal: A hamburger on a white bun and ice cream. I was very upset. How did they think he got clogged arteries in the first place?

Unfortunately, many people consider the opinion of their doctor higher than anything else, even higher than what they believe God can do. If your doctor tells you that you have terminal cancer and that there is no hope for recovery, what do you do? Get ready to die? If you believe your doctor, you probably will die. If you put all your trust in God, just wait and see what He can do. Why do we leave God out? Or only seek Him when all else fails?

It is better to trust in the LORD than to put confidence in man. Psalm 118:8

Commit thy way unto the LORD; trust also in Him; and He shall bring it to pass. Psalm 37:5

Trust in Him at all times; ye people, pour out your heart before Him: God is a refuge for us. Psalm 62:8

Are you including God in all your decisions? If a medical doctor prescribes a medication or recommends surgery, do you just take his word that this is the best thing for you? These are things you need to pray about and ask God for His perfect advice about. After making a decision like that, do you get a sense of peace or do you have a sense of unsettlement? Ask God what direction He would have you go. He may send you to another doctor. He may tell you to change your diet. He may instruct you to change your attitude or lifestyle.

God has His hand in all that we do, if we allow Him. The Bible instructs us to seek Him first. He wants us to totally rely upon Him. He wants us to listen to the prompting of the Holy Spirit. When eating that piece of chocolate cake or having that second serving of ice cream or that third donut, do you ever get the feeling that "you don't need that" or "don't eat that"? So, why did you? That's the prompting of the Holy Spirit trying to tell you something. If you don't pay attention to Him, eventually He is going to stop talking to you and He is likely to get your attention in another way that will make you very sorry you did not listen.

God wants our full attention. We are to *Pray without ceasing* (1 Thessalonians 5:17) — to be in constant communion with Him. When we are, He will instruct us as to what we should and should not do in all aspects of our life and health.

God wants us to rely upon Him not just on a daily basis, but on a minute-by-minute basis. He wants us to rely upon Him, not ourselves... *Trust in the LORD with all thine heart; and lean not unto thine own understanding* (Proverbs 3:5) ... and no one else. It doesn't matter what their credentials are – M.D., Ph.D., D.O., D.C., and don't believe me either. Look in the scriptures and seek your own answers. If you are sincere in your desire to know God's will, He will tell you everything you need to know. Note that I did not say, "God will tell you everything." God will tell you everything *He thinks you need to know.*

Melvin wrote:

> *In December of 1988 I developed some breathing problems. One doctor I saw said it was asthma. In January 1989, another doctor prescribed a 10-day course of Prednisone, an anti-inflammatory steriod. During that time, my breathing improved, but after I stopped taking the Prednisone, my problems returned. The doctor put me back on the steroid, but as soon as I stopped, my breathing problems would start up again. This "on and off" went on for all of 1989. It was a very difficult year; I couldn't do any physical work as I just couldn't shake the breathing problem. I just couldn't seem to get off this drug, even though I had heard it was really hard on your bones and other parts of the body to take it all the time. I was taking 40 mg. a day. The doctor knew it was bad for me too, but thought I should continue taking it anways.*
>
> *In January of 1990, I ended up in the hospital in Pelican Rapids. That doctor referred me to the Mayo Clinic. (I also found out that anyone can make an appointment at the Mayo Clinic, which I never knew.)*

The Mayo Clinic doctor told me I couldn't con-tinue going on and off Prednisone. I leveled off tak-ing 15-20 mg. a day. I did this for five years, and it did allow me to work. The Prednisone may have helped my breathing, but it does have side effects. One of these was that it interfered with my sleep, and I could only sleep a few hours a night, but this gave me a lot of time to read the scriptures.

In 1994, the Mayo Clinic doctor suggested I slowly taper off the Prednisone and prescribed a nebulizer treatment with Lydocaine. This treatment took 20 minutes four times a day. I used this time to search and study the scriptures. In about two months, I was off of the Prednosine,

Psalm 119 says: I have declared my ways, and thou heardest me: teach me thy statutes. Make me to understand the way of thy precepts: so shall I talk of thy wondrous works. My soul melteth for heaviness: strengthen thou me according unto thy word. Remove from me the way of lying: and grant me thy law graciously. I have chosen the way of truth: thy judgments have I laid before me. I have stuck unto thy testimonies: O LORD, put me not to shame. I will run the way of thy commandments, when thou shalt enlarge my heart. Teach me, O LORD, the way of thy statutes; and I shall keep it unto the end. Give me understanding, and I shall keep thy law; yea, I shall observe it with my whole heart. Make me to go in the path of thy command-ments; for therein do I delight. (26-35)

Over time, I was able to taper down on the

nebulizer treatment to once per day. Eventually, I was able to skip a day and so on.

In October of 2000, I went in for a checkup and was told I no longer had the need for any medication! Praise God!

I know that the Lord directed me to a doctor that cared more about my long-term health, not just in relieving my symptoms. It is important to realize that the doctors we go to for advice work for us. We are not required to do what they say. This seems to have gotten turned around somehow and many people think they have to do what they say. It's not so.

In looking back on my health struggles, I can see how many, many things the Lord wanted to show me. I was reading and studying the scriptures when I was in the military, but after I got married, I somehow got away from it. He really opened my eyes.

...Before I was afflicted I went astray: but now have I kept thy word. Thou art good, and doest good; teach me thy statutes. The proud have forged a lie against me: but I will keep thy precepts with my whole heart. (Psalm 119: 67-69)

...Unless thy law had been my delights, I should then have perished in mine affliction. I will never forget thy precepts: for with them thou hast quickened me. I am thine, save me; for I have sought thy precepts. The wicked have waited for me to destroy me: but I will consider thy testimonies. I have seen an end of all perfection: but thy commandment is exceeding broad. O how love I thy law! it is my meditation all the day. (Psalm 119: 92-97)

God Works in Mysterious Ways

Tess was a precocious eight year old when she heard her parents talking about her little brother, Andrew. All she knew was that he was very sick and they were completely out of money. They were moving to an apartment complex next month because they didn't have the money for the doctor bills and the house.

Only a very costly surgery could save him now and it was looking like there was no-one to loan them the money. She heard Daddy say to her tearful Mother with whispered desperation, "Only a miracle can save him now."

Tess went to her bedroom and pulled a glass jelly jar from its hiding place in the closet. She poured all the change out on the floor and counted it carefully, three times. The total had to be exactly perfect. No chance here for mistakes. Carefully placing the coins back in the jar and twisting on the cap, she slipped out the back door and made her way six blocks to Rexall's Drug Store with the big red Indian Chief sign above the door. She waited patiently for the pharmacist to give her some attention but he was too busy at this moment. Tess twisted her feet to make a scuffing noise. Nothing. She cleared her throat with the most disgusting sound she could muster. No good.

Finally, she took a quarter from her jar and banged it on the glass counter. That did it!

"And what do you want?" the pharmacist asked in an annoyed tone of voice. "I'm talking to my brother from Chicago whom I haven't seen in ages,"" he said without waiting for a reply to his question.

"Well, I want to talk to you about my brother," Tess answered in the same annoyed tone. "He's really, really sick... and I want to buy a miracle."

"I beg your pardon?" said the pharmacist.

"His name is Andrew and he has something bad growing inside his head and my Daddy says only a miracle can save him now. So how much does a miracle cost?"

"We don't sell miracles here, little girl. I'm sorry but I can't help you," the pharmacist said, softening a little.

"Listen, I have the money to pay for it. If it isn't enough, I will get the rest. Just tell me how much it costs."

The pharmacist's brother was a well dressed man. He stooped down and asked the little girl, "What kind of a miracle does your brother need?"

"I don't know," Tess replied with her eyes welling up. "I just know he's really sick and Mommy says he needs an operation. But my Daddy can't pay for it, so I want to use my money."

"How much do you have?" asked the man from Chicago.

"One dollar and eleven cents," Tess answered barely audibly. "And it's all the money I have, but I can get some more if I need to."

"Well, what a coincidence," smiled the man. "A dollar and eleven cents — the exact price of a miracle for little brothers." He took her money in one hand and with the other hand he grasped her mitten and said "Take me to where you live. I want to see your brother and meet your parents. Let's see if I have the kind of miracle you need."

That well-dressed man was Dr. Carlton Armstrong, a surgeon, specializing in neuro-surgery. The operation was completed without charge and it wasn't long until Andrew was home again and doing well. Mom and Dad were happily talking about the chain of events that had led them to this place. "That surgery," her Mom whispered, "was a real miracle. I wonder how much it would have cost?"

Tess smiled. She knew exactly how much a miracle cost... one dollar and eleven cents – plus the faith of a little child. A miracle is not the suspension of natural law, but the operation of a higher law.

And The Drugs...

I have made it clear how *I* feel about drugs, but let us examine what the scriptures have to say about the use of pharmaceutical drugs.

The word *pharmacy* comes from the Greek words *pharmakeia* and *pharmakeus* defined from Strongs:

Pharmakeia (Greek 5331) {far-mak-i'-ah}: sorcery 2, witchcraft 1; 3

1) the use or the administering of drugs

2) poisoning

3) sorcery, magical arts, often found in connection with idolatry and fostered by it

4) metaphor- the deceptions and seductions of idolatry

Pharmakeus (Greek 5332) {far-mak-yoos'} from pharmakon (a drug, i.e. spell-giving potion); A druggist "pharmacist" or poisoner: sorcerer 1; 1

1) one who prepares or uses magical remedies

2) sorcerer

There are several scriptures which use these Greek terms - all clearly describing the use of these things as sin: *Now the works of the flesh are manifest, which are these; Adultery, fornication, uncleanness, lasciviousness, Idolatry,* **witchcraft (Greek 5331),** *hatred, variance, emulations, wrath, strife, seditions, heresies.* Galatians 5:19-20

> *But the fearful, and unbelieving, and the abominable, and murderers, and whoremongers, and* **sorcerers (Greek 5332),** *and idolaters, and all liars, shall have their part in the lake which burneth with fire and brimstone: which is the second death.* Revelations 21:8

God designed the physical body with an incredible ability to continually renew and heal itself.

> *I will praise thee; for I am fearfully and wonderfully made: marvellous are thy works; and that my soul knoweth right well.* Psalms 139:14

HEALTH PROTECTIVE PROPERTIES IN OUR FOODS

God's Preventative Medicine: Phytochemicals

Garlic contains **allylic sulfides:** Inhibits cholesterol synthesis and protects against carcinogens and **canima-glutamylallylic cysteines:** May have a role in lowering blood pressure, and elevating immune system activities.

Flaxseed, soy products, purslane and **walnuts** contain **alpha-linolenic acid:** Reduces inflammation and stimulates the immune system.

Parsley, carrots, winter squash, sweet potatoes, yams, cantaloupe, apricots, spinach, kale, turnip greens and **citrus fruits** contain **carotenoids:** Antioxidant that protects against cancer and may help reduce accumulation of arterial plaque.

Green tea and **berries** contain **catechins:** Protect against gastrointestinal cancer; may aid the immune system and lower cholesterol.

Parsley, carrots and **citrus fruits** contain **coumarins:** Prevents blood clotting and may have anti-cancer activity.

Parsley, carrots, broccoli, cabbage, cucumbers, squash, yams, tomatoes, egg-plant, peppers, mint, basil and **citrus fruits** contain **monoterpenes:** Cancer-fighting antioxidants that inhibit cholesterol production and aids protective enzyme activity.

Cabbage, brussels sprouts and **kale** contain **indoles:** Induce protective enzymes that deactivate estrogen.

Squash, yams, tomatoes, eggplant, peppers, soy products and **berries** contain **flavonoids:** Block receptor sites for certain hormones involved in cancer promotion.

Mustard, horseradish and **radishess** contain **Isothiniocyanates:** Powerful inducers of protective enzymes.

Citrus fruits contain **limonoids**: Powerful inducers of protective enzymes.

Tomatoes and **red grapefruit** contain **lycopene:** Powerful carotenoid antioxidant that helps the body resist cancer and its progression.

Parsley, carrots, broccoli, cabbage, tomatoes, eggplant, peppers, citrus fruits, whole grains and **berries** contain **phenolic acids:** May help the body resist cancer by inhibiting nitrosamine formation and affecting enzymes.

Parsley, carrots and **celery** contain **Phthalides:** Stimulate the production of beneficial enzymes that detoxify carcinogens.

Broccoli, cabbage, cucumbers, squash, sweet potatoes, yams, tomatoes, eggplant, peppers, soy products and **whole grains** contain **plant sterols:** Block estrogen promotion of breast cancer activity, help block the absorption of cholesterol.

Citrus fruit, licorice-root extract and **soy products** contain **triterpenoids:** Prevents dental decay and acts as an anti-ulcer agent. Binds to estrogen and inhibits cancer by suppressing unwanted enzyme activity.

If we cut ourselves, the tissues are able to mend themselves. If we are exposed to a bacteria or virus, the immune system sends white blood cells to identify, kill and dispose of such undesirables (and also potentially cancerous cells, cellular debris, etc.) in the body. We may suffer some symptoms (runny nose, congestion, headache, fever, diarrhea, etc.) while this happens, but if the immune system is healthy, we will recover.

Man has created all sorts of chemical remedies (drugs) to mask these cold and flu symptoms, but they don't help heal the body in any way. In fact, they may slow down the body's ability to heal itself and have many dangerous side effects. One manufacture of over-the-counter allergy and cold remedies has recently withdrawn all of their products containing Phenylpropanolamine (PPA) which the FDA recently reported to be linked to increased hemorrhagic stroke (bleeding in brain) and seizures. This drug (which is also found in weight control products as an appetite suppressent) has been available for years.

We know it is always better to solve the root problem than to mask the symptoms. There are some drugs which are lifesavers. The problem seems to lie upon the daily use and reliance of pharmaceutical drugs.

God's perfect plan is not really to heal us but to not have us get sick in the first place. There is overwhelming scientific evidence that the body can protect and heal itself more effectively if we take care of the body through proper nutritional support, avoidance of pollutants and toxins, moderate lifestyle, adequate rest, fresh air and physical activity.

What About Diet?

There is no question in my mind that we have a responsibility to treat our bodies as a holy temple. We need to avoid the things that do not support good health and provide proper nourishment for our bodies through the foods we eat. The foundation for my previous books on nutrition have been based on the principals in the following two scriptures:

Know ye not that ye are the temple of God, and that the Spirit of God dwelleth in you? If any man defile the temple of God, him shall God destroy; for the temple of God is holy, which temple ye are. 1 Corinthians 3:16-17

Whether therefore ye eat, or drink, or whatsoever ye do, do all to the glory of God. 1 Corinthians 10:31

This is the fundamental principle of practical godliness. Nothing must be done against the glory of God, and the good of those around us. In whatever we do, we should keep God in mind in what He would have us do.

Matthew Henry writes, *Our own appetite must not*

determine our practice, but the honour of God and the good and edification of the church. We should not so much consult our own pleasure and interest as the advancement of the kingdom of God among men.

What does the Bible say about diet? Quite a bit actually. Sometimes, it may be difficult to determine what guidelines given in the Old Testament apply to the law, and what applies to today under the new covenant. Peter's dream in Acts clearly tells us that the foods which were deemed unclean in Levisicus were acceptable to eat.

> Upon the which when I had fastened mine eyes, I considered, and saw four-footed beasts of the earth, and wild beasts, and creeping things, and fowls of the air. And I heard a voice saying unto me, Arise, Peter; slay and eat. But I said, Not so, Lord: for nothing common or unclean hath at any time entered into my mouth. But the voice answered me again from heaven, What God hath cleansed, that call not thou common. And this was done three times: and all were drawn up again into heaven. Acts 11:6-10

Note that *this was done three times*. This demonstrates the significance of what God was trying to show Peter.

> All things are lawful unto me, but all things are not expedient (beneficial): all things are lawful for me, but I will not be brought under the power of any. Meats for the belly, and the belly for meats: but God shall destroy both it and them. 1 Corinthians 6:12-13

There is a tremendous amount of dietary wisdom in the Bible. Much of the information given in Leviticus Chapter 11 is under the Old Testament Law given to preserve the sanctity of Israel as God's holy people. However, God is not without reason. These guidelines may also have been for important health considerations.

And the priest shall burn them upon the altar: it is the food of the offering made by fire for a sweet savour: all the fat is the LORD's. It shall be a perpetual statute throughout your generations in all your dwellings, that ye shall eat neither fat nor blood. Leviticus 3:16-17

Say to the Israelites: 'Do not eat any of the fat of cattle, sheep or goats. The fat of an animal found dead or torn by wild animals may be used for any other purpose, but you must not eat it.' Leviticus 7:23-24 (NIV)

It is important to realize that salvation is not based upon our dietary choices. According to scripture, we have a new covenant (through Christ) which was established upon better promises (Hebrews 8:6-12), so therefore, today, we cannot say that it is a sin to eat fat or the blood, but it is for our own good that we do not (Acts 15:19). God states that what He has cleansed let no man call unclean (Acts 10:9-21; Acts 11:1-18; Romans 14). This does not negate the fact that God has clearly laid down some important dietary guidelines that would be helpful for us all – even today, to sustain a very long and healthy life. Our health, on the other hand, is based upon our dietary choices.

Leviticus 11 tells us which animals could or could not be eaten (under the law). The grounds for the prohibition was that the fat was the richest part of the animal, and therefore belonged to God (Leviticus 3:16). Fat stood as the sign of healthfulness and vigor, and referred to the the richest and choicest specimens or examples of the animal. It was also part of an important teaching that the idea of self-denial, and the maxim that the richest and best meat of the edible animal belonged to God.

The law was probably also a sanitary restriction, for, at an early date, leprosy, scrofula and disfiguring cutaneous diseases were thought to be caused by the use of fat as food. Most diseases were transferred through the blood and the fat of animals.

Blood is considered the bearer of life (Leviticus 17:14). Acts 15:19 also states that we should not eat the blood from meat. *That ye abstain from meats offered to idols, and from blood, and from things strangled, and from fornication: from which if ye keep yourselves, ye shall do well. Fare ye well.*

God has our best interests in mind at all times. If we take a look at all of the major health problems that exist today, we can see how the principals God gave us prevent problems associated with excess intake of fat and food:

Obesity
Heart disease
Diabetes
Cancer

The Sin of Overeating, Gluttony, and Rich Foods

The sin of indulgence of the appetite in eating and drinking is mentioned several times in the Bible. *When thou sittest to eat with a ruler, consider diligently what is before thee: And put a knife to thy throat, if thou be a man given to appetite. Be not desirous of his dainties: for they are deceitful meat* (Proverbs 23:1-3). We must restrain ourselves into moderation, from all excess.

Be not among winebibbers; among riotous eaters of flesh: For the drunkard and the glutton shall come to poverty: and drowsiness shall clothe a man with rags. Proverbs 23:20-21

Our focus on food had become corrupt. Yes, food can be enjoyed. The problem stems from the overindulgance and misuse. Instead of eating when we are hungry and stopping when we are full, we stuff ourselves to the point of discomfort and eat when we are bored, depressed, stessed, lonely, and even out of simple habit. Some people are just simply addicted to food.

Looking in the refrigerator for comfort, to calm us down after a stressful day, to raise our spirits if we feel depressed or bored, and any other time than when you feel hungry is wrong. It is sinful to look to *anything* other than God for our hope and solutions. Obsession with food is no more acceptable to God than alcoholism or drug addiction is to Him.

John 6:41 states, *I am the bread which came down*

from heaven. Verse 58 continues, *he that eateth of this bread shall live for ever.*

He reminds them of the Isrealites in the desert and their obsession with what they would eat. *This is that bread which came down from heaven: not as your fathers did eat manna and are dead* (John 6:58). *It is the spirit that quickeneth; the flesh profiteth nothing: the words that I speak unto you, they are spirit, and they are life* (John 6:63). It is clear that our focus is not to be on fleshly concerns – as God will provide. We are to place our focus on things of the spirit.

It is estimated that 100 million Americans are above their ideal weight. Obesity, defined as weighing over 20% of your ideal weight, is a major nutritional obstacle in America today, reaching epidemic status. More than one-third of all adults and one in five children are considered obese. Each year, obesity causes at least 300,000 excess deaths in the U.S. and costs the country more than $133 billion on healthcare, diets and diet-related products – and we are still fat. We are even slower than the Isrealites!

While overeating is not the only reason for weight problems, it certainly plays a significant role. Many people take great pleaure in simply stuffing themselves at mealtime, going to all-you-can-eat buffets for one helping after another or eating an entire bag of chips or cookies in one sitting. I really can't picture Jesus at a buffet pigging out or even eating at a fast food place. If we claim we are Christians, how is this behavior for us Christ-like? Paul's second letter to Timothy stresses that we need to deny ourselves of the physical pleasures of the world. *If we believe not, yet he abideth faith-ful: he cannot deny himself* (Timothy 2:13).

And he said to them all, If any man will come after me, let him deny himself, and take up his cross daily, and follow me. Luke 9:23

The reason for fasting is not for weight control, but did you realise that if you fasted for one day a week for a year, you would be consuming approximately 106,000 fewer calories. One pound is equivalent to 3,500 calories, so the potential to lose over 30 pounds exists (providing you don't make up for the loss on the other days).

The spiritual benefits of fasting are so awesome – allowing such a personal intimacy with God so He can really work in your life – the weight-control benefits are just part of the built-in wisdom of our all-knowing Lord.

Food Choices

A major reason for health problems and excess weight is poor food choices and malnutrition. We eat too much processed foods with low nutrient value – "junk food." These foods literally provide "empty calories" – little or no nutritional value other than the calories they provide. But, if we cannot use these calories, they are readily stored as fat. Refined foods lack the nutrients required for efficient energy production and tremendously increase the body's requirement for them. Unrefined foods (the way God made them!) naturally contain these nutrients (B Vitamins, Vitamin C, chromium, magnesium, manganese and other trace minerals), but they are lost in processing.

When there is inadequate intake of all essential nutrients, fat is not efficiently burned. Fat is burned only if sufficient energy is produced. Energy production depends on almost every known nutrient, especially the B Vitamins. Fat is burned at a greatly reduced rate if B-5 and protein are under supplied. Vitamin B6 is necessary for the energy conversion of stored fat.

Vitamin E is necessary for fat utilization. Sufficient amounts of E actually doubles our ability to use fat. Lecithin aids the cells to burn fat. If we are deficient in the nutrients necessary for fat metabolism, poor fat utilization results. Instead, the fat is stored.

Added pounds are accompanied by increases in blood pressure, blood fat and blood sugar. Overweight individuals are more prone to cancer (most specifically, breast and endometrial), heart disease, kidney disease, diabetes, high blood pressure, malnutrition, liver disorders, gall bladder disorders, respiratory problems, arthritis, gout, complications of pregnancy, psychological problems and more.

High Blood Pressure

Hypertension, or high blood pressure, is primarily caused by a combination of dietary factors and genetics. Obesity is a primary factor of high blood pressure. Achieving ideal body weight has demonstrated to nearly normalize blood pressure of many overweight individuals. For every 10% increase in body weight, blood pressure rises 6.5mm/Hg. Other common associated problems include: Hardening of the arteries and fluid buildup (edema), due to sodium retention or mineral imbalances.

Too Much Salt!

The intake of excess sodium is a huge problem, especially in the United States. In the last 100 years, we have experienced a 20-fold increase in our intake of sodium. This was accompanied by about a one–third drop in potassium intake.

We have been spoiled by eating our potatoes with salt, butter, and sour cream, or worse yet, deep fried and salted. It may take a little adjusting as we introduce our taste buds to foods in their natural form, instead of hiding them under fat and salt. Soon you won't miss a thing and you will grow to appreciate their real taste.

Obesity and a high salt diet often go hand in hand. High blood pressure is virtually nonexistent in primitive societies that consume diets which are low in salt and high in potassium. The intake of sodium chloride (table salt) is horrendous. Sodium in this form is difficult for the body to get rid of, and it is easily retained.

High sodium intake increases the loss of potassium and magnesium and possibly some calcium. It is difficult to detect a potassium deficiency because the blood will draw it from other sources in the body to maintain a normal level, resulting in abdominal bloating, fatigue, mental fuzziness, physical weakness, even nausea, light headedness and high blood pressure, etc.

In 1988 in a federal health and nutrition survey, people who consumed less than 1,200 mg (the average intake of potassium) of potassium per day had twice the incidence of hypertension as people who consumed 3,600 mg. per day.

An extra 400 mg. of potassium (a glass of orange

juice or a generous slice of cantaloupe) daily can reduce risk of stroke-related death by 40%. High potassium levels help block the sodium absorption by the kidneys. Potassium acts as a natural diuretic, lowering the volume of blood plasma and decreases blood pressure.

While we should consume no more than 2,000 mg. sodium per day, the average consumption is between 5,000-15,000 mg. Americans consume over four times more salt than the average intake from all other countries round the world!

Sodium Chloride Content of Food Items:

Salt (1 tsp): **2,132 mg.**
McDonald's Quarter Pounder w/Cheese: **1,150 mg.**
Hardee's Big Country Breakfast: **2,870 mg.**
Hormel Chili (15 oz.): **1,127 mg.**
Frozen Microwave Pizza, saus./cheese (7.5oz.): **1,300 mg.**
Pizza Hut, Pepperoni Personal Pan Pizza: **1,335 mg.**
Cambells Chunky Soups (8 oz.): **822 mg.**
Cambells Chicken Noodle Soup (10 oz.): **1,050 mg.**
Spaghetti with Sausage (2.5 cups): **2,437 mg.**
Linguini with Red Clam Sauce, (3 cups): **2,182 mg.**
Garlic Bread (8 oz.): **1,083 mg.**
Ham (3 oz.) and Swiss (1 oz.) Sandwich: **1,553 mg.**
Kraft Processed American Cheese (2 oz.): **890 mg.**
Green Beans, canned, Del Monte (1 cup): **925 mg.**
Dill pickle (1 large): **1,928 mg.**
Frozen Pancakes w/ Sausage (6 oz): **1,140 mg.**
Average sodium content for frozen meals: **1,175 mg.**

My favorite substitute for salt?
Lemon juice!

Cancer

Studies show an increased risk of breast and colorectal cancer risk with increased intake of refined carbohydrates such as sugar, bread and pasta, pork and processed meats and potatoes (breast cancer only), cakes and desserts (colon and rectum cancers only). Most vegetables were inversely associated with cancer of the colon and rectum, whereas only carrots and raw vegetables seemed to lower breast cancer risk. High fruit intake was associated only with a reduction of rectal cancer. Total energy intake was directly associated with all cancer sites. Among macronutrients, high intake of starch and saturated fat seemed to lead to an increase of cancer risk. High intakes of polyunsaturated fatty acids (chiefly derived from olive oil and seed oils) were cancer protective. Among micronutrients, beta-carotene, Vitamin E, and calcium showed inverse associations with breast and colorectal cancer risk. (Franceschi)

A high fat diet and obesity have been associated with increased risk of cancer at a number of sites, including endometrium, postmenopausal breast, kidney, colorectum, pancreas and prostate. (Guthrie)

Think this stuff is boring?

My people are destroyed for the lack of knowledge... Hosea 4:6

Diabetes

Obesity is associated with a greater risk of diabetes. Diabetes mellitus, whether insulin-dependent or non-insulin dependent, is a disease of carbohydrate metabolism. The majority of those with diabetes are non–insulin dependent. Many of these individuals are overweight or obese. It has been noted for over 50 years that glucose tolerance can be improved with a reduction in body weight.

Maintaining normal weight is also the primary factor in diabetes prevention. Avoidance of refined sugars not only helps keep your weight down, but it also very simply may prevent diabetes.

Simple carbohydrates in the form of refined sugar are quickly absorbed into the body causing a rapid increase in blood sugar (glucose). This causes the pancreas to respond with an outpouring of insulin to lower the amount of glucose by means of carrying it into the cells to be burned as fuel.

Natural unrefined foods such as grains, beans, vegetables, etc. contain fiber which has a slowing effect upon absorption rate. Complex carbohydrates take longer to break down into simple sugars and thus cause a more gradual release into the blood stream. This is far less stressful to the pancreas.

Heart Disease

Cardiovascular disease accounts for approximately 50% of all deaths in the United States. It is estimated that 65 million Americans have some form of heart or blood vessel disease at a cost of over $90 billion a year.

This review sums up the effects of a high fat diet pretty clearly:

"It has been found that regular intake of foods with saturated fats such as meat and certain dairy products raise the risk of coronary heart disease. The total mixed-fat intake is associated with a higher incidence of the nutritionally linked cancers, specifically cancer of the postmenopausal breast, distal colon, prostate, pancreas, ovary and endometrium. The associated genotoxic carcinogens for several of these cancers are heterocyclic amines, which also play a role in heart-disease causation, and these are produced during the broiling and frying of creatine-containing foods such as meats. Monounsaturated oils such as olive or canola oil are low-risk fats as shown in animal models and through the observation that the incidence of specific diseases is lower in the Mediterranean region, where such oils are customarily used. High salt intake is associated with high blood pressure and with stomach cancer, especially with inadequate intake of potassium from fruits and vegetables and of calcium from certain vegetables and low-fat dairy products. Vegetables, fruits and soy products are rich in antioxidants that are essential to lower disease risk stemming from reactive oxygen systems in the body."

Eat to live, not live to eat by JH Weisburger, American Health Foundation, Valhalla, New York, *Nutrition* 2000 Sep;16(9):767-73.

A number of dietary factors have a significant effect on coronary heart disease: Overeating and obesity, high fat intake and high cholesterol, high blood pressure and glucose intolerance.

Liver Damage

Liver problems are common among overweight persons, largely because of a high fat diet. The liver has the responsibility to metabolize the fat we eat. If it becomes overloaded, fat will accumulate in the liver tissue impairing its 500 other important functions such as producing enzymes, bile and hemoglobin, processing glucose, proteins, vitamins and most other compounds used by the body. The liver is also responsible for metabolizing alcohol, nicotine and any other poisons we ingest from our water, food or air.

A diet including complete proteins, the B Complex Vitamins, choline, Vitamins B12, C and E and lecithin aid the restoration of the liver.

Circulation Problems

Circulation problems such as varicose veins, hemorrhoids, hiatal hernias are commonly seen among individuals who are overweight. Constipation commonly accompanies the type of diet seen in overweight persons: high fat, low fiber. Constipation is often accompanied by varicose veins, hemorrhoids and hiatal hernias.

Other health problems associated with a high fat diet and being overweight include: Gout, gall stones (which are formed by cholesterol and bile), arthritis and gynecological irregularities.

Dying Young

Genesis 6:3 states, *And the LORD said, My spirit shall not always strive with man, for that he also is flesh: yet his days shall be an hundred and twenty years.*

At the height of the Roman Empire, people only lived to be about 26 years old. At the beginning of the 20th century the average life expectancy for a U.S. male was 49 years.

Improvements in public health in developed countries over the last two centuries have led to a recent dramatic increase in the average life expectancy at birth. Fewer people now die in childhood of infectious diseases and from the effect of poor diet. Nevertheless, even in the absence of disease, everybody ages, resulting in long term decline and eventual death. Typically, people die from this aging process between 70-80, though some people have sufficient strength to live longer (Psalm 90:10).

Today, the average life expectancy at birth in the U.S. is close to 80 years. In Japan, women can now expect to live to nearly 83.

The oldest known person, Sharali Misimiv, was believed to be 168 years old. He lived in a remote Russian village, where he died in 1973. The people of Abkhasia, the remote mountain region of southern Russia, were renowned for their longevity. Also from this area was the oldest known woman who reportedly died at age 140. In this area, most people are simple field workers where there are few paved roads and other amenities of modern living. They credit their good health to exercise and light eating.

Another community famed for their longevity are the Hunzas, who are said to live to be healthy, active and disease free, well past the age of 100. There are other communities like this as well. All of these communities base their living on simplicity and wholesome ness. Their lives are uncomplicated and void of the stress that dominates so many of our lives. Most of us in the U.S. would think that these people are a couple hundred years behind the times and also, very boring.

Some researchers suggest that the life expectancy of other animals can give us a rough idea of our own. The life expectancy of most other animals is roughly seven times the point at which they reach maturity. A medium size dog, for example, reaches full growth at around two years, the life expectancy is around 14. A horse reaches maturity about three, and lives to be 20-25. Rabbits can live to be seven years old, while they reach maturity at about 11 months. Hamsters live about five years and reach maturity at about eight months. Humans reach maturity around age 20. This, times seven equals 140 years. But many of us barely reach just half this age.

In 1997, the top causes of death were as follows:

1) Heart disease, 33%
2) Cancer, 23%
3) Strokes, 7%
4) Lung diseases, 4%
5) Accidents, 4%
6) Pneumonia/Flu, 4%
7) Diabetes, 2%
8) Suicide, 1.4%
9) AIDS, 1.4%
10) Liver disease/Cirrhosis, 1.2%

Almost every one of these can be largely prevented or at least postponed with proper diet and lifestyle habits. Alcohol use and abuse can contribute to heart disease, cancer, stroke, liver disease and even accidents. Smoking is a major contributor to many of these causes as well.

The quality of the time that we live is every bit as important as the length. We can do more to ensure a better quality of life as we age. Nearly 60% of all people over 65 years have high blood pressure, and nearly one-third have heart disease. Forty-five percent of the elderly are on prescription drugs for arthritis, hypertension, glaucoma, etc.

Eat Less, Live Longer

According to Roy Walford, researcher and author of *The 120-Year Diet*, we could plan on living 30 to 50 years longer than we originally expected if we consumed less calories, a lot less calories.

A number of studies have shown that the life span of animals can be extended by restricting their food intake. Rats fed 40% fewer calories lived 50% longer than their unrestricted peers. That corresponds to humans living to be 150-160 years old.

Walford and a number of others have shown that cutting calories in young animals delays a loss of heart muscle function that ordinarily occurs with aging, and can extend the reproductive years. Fewer calories keep their immune systems from deteriorating with age.

Walford and associates reported in the 1992

Proceeding for The National Academy of Sciences that a calorically restricted (average of 1,780 kcal/day), low-fat (10% of calories), nutrient-dense diet in humans has a large number of health benefits. The diet significantly lowers weight in men and women, lowers blood glucose, lowers total leukocyte count, reduces cholesterol levels and decreases blood pressure.

William Castelli, director of the famous Framingham Heart Study which monitored the health of thousands of residents of the city near Boston since 1958, reports that in Framingham, Massachusetts, those who weigh between 11-20% below the average weight for their height have the lowest risk of early death. Other researchers have also demonstrated the effect of caloric restriction on age-associated cancers.

Enhanced Immune Response

Animal studies show that low calorie diets have a positive effect upon immunity. Walford and his associates demonstrated that dietary restriction enhanced immunity to an infectious agent, influenza, as well as enhanced other immunologic parameters. Dietary restriction significantly inhibited the normal age-related decline in immune responses.

Enhanced Use of Insulin

Walford and other researchers also investigated the relationship of aging and restriction of dietary calories upon insulin. In this study they found that reducing calories by 52% extends maximum life span by approximately 33% and increases insulin receptors by 15% to

25%. Increased insulin receptors allow us to more efficiently use the energy from the food we eat.

Reduced dietary calories, enhanced nutrient intakes, and modification of fatty acids benefited patients with non-insulin-dependent diabetes mellitus (NIDDM) in a study with 86 obese subjects (aged 40-64) with recently diagnosed NIDDM. In this study, the patients undergoing dietary therapy resulted in greater weight loss, better metabolic control and an improved blood lipid profile than the control.

While many diabetics are aware of the need to limit simple sugars, most do not limit their intake of dietary fat or increase their intake of high fiber foods, which are also necessary to obtain ideal weight and stable blood sugar levels.

Free Radical Protection

Oxidation is part of the natural metabolic process of the body. When fatty acids are burned as fuel for the body, oxidation occurs, which produces free radicals. In humans the level of oxidative DNA damage can be lessened by caloric restriction and dietary composition. Less food eaten means less oxidation and fewer free radicals produced. (Simic)

The basic mechanisms of aging and its retardation by caloric restriction remain unclear. Reducing calories may retard aging based on the reduced production of mitochondrial free radicals. (Feuers) The less food we consume, the less work it is for the body to process and metabolise it - burning calories produces free radicals.

Improved Inflammatory Conditions

Inflammatory conditions such as arthritis, psoriasis, allergies, etc, are very difficult to treat successfully. It is known that imbalances of inflammatory and anti inflammatory hormones contribute to the problem.

Caloric restriction may also help reduce production of a powerful inflammatory component (Interleukin-6 or IL-6) in the body. Blood levels of IL-6 are normally very low – usually non-detectable in the absence of inflammation. As we grow older, however, the levels increase. (Ershler)

Researchers also speculate that IL-6 may contribute to the development of several degenerative diseases that are common in late-life including arthritis, lymphoma, osteoporosis and Alzheimer's disease. This age-related process can be largely prevented by life span-extending dietary restriction. (Ershler)

Reduce Risk Factors for Heart Disease

Obesity is a risk factor for the development of heart disease. Weight reduction is an effective long-term therapy for maintaining normal blood pressure. (Davis).

Researchers (Singh and associates) found that dietary strategies are highly effective to reduce other risk factors associated with cardiovascular diseases. To study the role of diet in cardiovascular risk-factor intervention, 458 high-risk individuals were asked to eat a cardiovaso-protective diet (high in complex carbohydrates, vegetable protein, fiber, Vitamin C, potassium and magnesium). Fats consumed consist largely of polyunsaturated fats, avoiding saturated fat and cholesterol. Total fat should be no more than 20% of the total caloric intake. After one year, there was a significant decrease in total risk factors:

1. Significant reduction in blood cholesterol.

2. Reduced blood pressure.

3. Reduced weight and modification of other risk factors and complications in patients with risk factors of coronary heart disease.

A Few Simple Rules:

1. Eat foods in their natural wholesome state (organic, if possible). Avoid processed, prepackaged, and "fast" foods. These are generally low in nutritional value and fiber, and often high in sodium and fat.

2. Drink lots of water.

3. Eat less, don't stuff yourself. It is far better to eat small meals often, rather than a few large meals daily. Always eat breakfast. This increases your metabolic rate all day.

4. Eat when you are hungry - at mealtime, not because you are bored, depressed or stressed.

5. Maintain an active lifestyle.

The Sin of Excess Sugar and Sweets

> *It is not good to eat much honey: so for men to search their own glory is not glory.* Proverbs 25:27

> *When thou sittest to eat with a ruler, Consider diligently him that is before thee; And put a knife to thy throat, If thou be a man given to appetite. Be not desirous of his dainties; Seeing they are deceitful meat.* Proverbs 23:1-3

In 1900, sugar consumption was 1-5 lbs. per person per year. Now, it is 150 lbs.

Sugar is much like a drug. It has addictive properties and adverse side effects. Sugar is not a whole natural food that does not even resemble the original sources that God made - sugar cane and sugar beets. Sugar is highly refined, fragmented, denatured, and completely stripped of all nutrients which were present in its original form. Sugar cane and sugar beets are natural and contain minerals, vitamins, trace elements, enzymes, essential fatty acids, amino acids, and very important FIBER. The final processed result is a pure crystallized form of sucrose, a white "pharmaceutically pure" chemical.

Compared to sugar, honey could practically be considered health food because honey does contain several minerals and nutrients to assist in the body's use of the carbohydrate, yet the Bible clearly warns us not to eat too much honey (Proverbs 25:27).

Concerning this verse, Matthew Henry writes that the pleasures of the sense (flesh) is something we must be graciously dead to. Though honey *pleases the taste, and, if eaten with moderation, is very wholesome, yet, if eaten to excess, it becomes nauseous, creates bile, and is the occasion of many diseases. It is true of all the delights of the children of men that they will surfeit, but never satisfy, and they are dangerous to those that allow themselves the liberal use of them.* (Henry)

Other than calories, sugar provides absolutely no nutritional value for our essential dietary needs. Sugar has no fiber, no vitamins, no minerals, no essential fatty acids, no antioxidants and no phytochemicals. To make matters worse, your body must tap into its precious supply of essential nutrients in order to process this highly refined chemical. In effect, sugar's empty calories double your nutrient deficit. Laboratory animals fed sugar die significantly sooner than animals fed the same number of calories as complex carbohydrates such as whole grains and beans.

Interestingly, in the processing of raw sugar cane or sugar beets, over 90% of the naturally-occurring chromium is lost. Chromium is needed for insulin to bring glucose into the cells to be used as fuel. Without chromium, we can not burn these calories, so instead, they are converted to fat and stored.

In addition to causing weight problems, sugar is a major contributing factor in the growth of many degenerative conditions such as diabetes, heart disease, tooth decay, periodontal disease and osteoporosis. Sugar consumption has also been associated with hyperactivity in children and criminal behavior.

Upon eating sugar-containing foods, the sugar is rapidly absorbed into the bloodstream raising the level of sugar in the blood to a dangerously high level. At this point one will feel an abundance of energy. This places inordinate stress on the pancreas as it is forced to compensate by producing and releasing high amounts of insulin which allows the sugar to enter the cells so it can be burned. The liver is also stressed as it must transform the sugar (unless we are running a marathon that day) to glycogen in order to store it. The adrenal glands, which are stimulated to increase their output of adrenaline, are also stressed.

The excess insulin not only rapidly brings the sugar level down, it lowers it *far below normal.* The term associated with this is *hypoglycemia or low blood sugar* causing fatigue, irritability, headaches and confusion. (This is often referred to as *the crash.*)

Many adults have poor insulin function. Normal amounts of insulin are produced, but because of the high-sugar diet, it is present more often than not. The cells eventually become less sensitive to this continual presence of insulin. Like the first few times the fire alarm goes off, we jump in response to it, but if it continually keeps ringing, we eventually ignore it.

Americans consume a huge amount of sugar – 40 teaspoons each day. Most of it, about 75%, is hidden in processed foods. In fact, sugar is the most commonly used food additive.

The top two sugar sources are soft drinks and commercial breakfast cereals, which also happen to be the two best-selling foods in America. Beef is third. Other major sugar sources are candy, ice cream and desserts.

The nine teaspoons of sugar in just one can of soda supplies 180 calories, almost 10% of the daily calorie requirement for an adult. Sugar accounts for an average of 640 calories per day or 24% of total calories, more than half of the carbohydrate content of the standard American diet.

Many people find sugar addictive. The more they eat, the more they crave it, and the more they must consume to satisfy their cravings.

We all know that candy and desserts contain sugar, but do you realize how much? Sugar is also often found in many surprising places: salt, peanut butter, bread, fruit juices, instant oatmeal, meat products, canned vegetables, mayonnaise, toothpaste, baby food, etc. Look how much is hiding in these popular foods:

Estimated teaspoons of sugar <u>per</u> <u>serving:</u>

Soda or pop (12 oz.)	9-10
Hard candy (4 oz.)	10
Apple or pumpkin pie (1 slice)	12
Sherbet (1/2 cup)	9
Flavored yogurt (8 oz.)	7
Koolaid (8 oz.)	6
Donut (glazed)	6
Ice cream (4 oz.)	5
Orange marmalade (1 tbsp.)	5
Canned corn (5 oz.)	3

General Mills Honey Nut Cheerios (2/3 cup) . 2.5

Kellogg's Fruitiful or Raisin Bran (2/3 cup) . 2.25

General Mills Raisin Nut Bran (2/3 cup) 2

Ketchup (1 tbsp.) 1

NOTE: Many manufactures try to "hide" sugar by giving it other names; corn syrup, corn syrup solids, maple syrup, molasses, cane syrup, fructose, dextrose, maltose, lactose, etc.

Did you know the entire blood volume of a typical adult contains the equivalent of only **5 teaspoons** *glucose (sugar)?*

Research has implicated excessive sugar consumption in the following health problems:

- Heart Disease
- Cancer
- Depression
- Diabetes
- Diverticulitis
- Urinary infections
- Gout
- High blood pressure
- Hormonal disorders
- Hypoglycemia
- Indigestion
- Kidney stones
- Mental & nervous disorders
- Migraine headaches
- Nutrient deficiencies
- Obesity
- Osteoporosis
- Periodontal disease
- Tooth decay

Sugar Turns to Fat

All simple sugars are rapidly digested and absorbed, and unless you quickly burn them off through exercise, are converted to fat. Acetates from sugar are the basic building blocks from which cholesterol, saturated fatty acids and triglycerides are made.

The more sugar (or other refined carbohydrates) you consume, the more acetate molecules you'll have in your system to support the production of saturated fat and cholesterol (and cellulite!). Sugar literally becomes fat. This fat is stored – well, you know where. It not only looks unattractive, but contributes to hardening of the arteries, heart attacks and many other health problems listed on the previous page.

Complex carbohydrates are burned much more slowly, and therefore do not trigger fat production.

Soda Pop

The consumption of soft drinks (pop) in both adults and children is incredible. Instead of water, juice and other healthy beverages, many people are now more commonly drinking soda, creating numerous serious health problems. (Guenther)

While the sugar content in soda is a major factor contributing to obesity and dental problems, even more of a health concern is the phosphoric acid content. Many people will switch from regular soda to diet sodas thinking that the sugar content is the cause of the dental problems they are experiencing, but the more serious culprit is phosphoric acid, aspartame and other dietary acids found in soda pop, especially colas. (Hughes)

Studies show an increase in calcium loss in postmenopausal women, the group which is already at the highest risk for the development for osteoporosis. Women who have a higher consumption of phosphoric acid-containing soft drinks tend to show increased serum levels of PTH and elevated phosphorus levels. Consumption of one or more bottles per day of cola soft drinks showed a clear association with low calcium levels. (Mazariegos-Ramos, Fernando)

Carbonated beverage consumption is also associated with increased bone fractures in younger individuals – including teenage girls. (Wyshak)

Over 100 published papers have reported the health-related damages or benefits in clinical or experimental studies. Harmful effects related to soft drink consumption included cavities and other dental disorders, mineral metabolism disorders, acid-peptic disease, other acid-base imbalance disturbances, urinary stone disease, hypocalcemia and increased risk for osteoporosis, neoplasm, risk factors for cardiovascular disease, effects on the central nervous system, reproduction, allergy and etc. (Amato, Shuster, Mazariegos-Ramos)

Loss of calcium is not just a problem for adult women. Calcium concentrations in children were compared to controls to assess whether the intake of at least 1.5 liters per week of soft drinks demonstrated a significant risk factor for the development of low calcium levels. The phosphoric acid they contain is very detrimental to our calcium stores. (Mazariegos-Ramos)

Animal studies suggest that the impact may even be more detrimental to younger individuals. (Amato)

Another problem associated with soft drinks is the fluoride they contain. Fluoride is an extremely hazardous substance that critically impairs many body functions. We have been told that it is good for us as it fights tooth decay, and therefore this known poison is deliberately added to our water supplies. We also add fluoride to toothpaste, mouthwash, medications, pesticides, herbicides, foods and beverages.

Excessive fluoride intake can cause skin eruptions, collagen breakdown, headaches, gastric distress, immune system weakness, reproductive problems, genetic damage, kidney disease, hip fractures in the elderly, heart problems, cancer and dental fluorosis. Dental fluorosis occurs as a result of excessive total fluoride intake during tooth development. This is an increasing problem as many children may receive substantial fluoride intake from soft drinks. (Heilman)

Fluoride levels of soda products tested averaged 0.72 ppm. Fluoride levels are not marked on soft drink product labels and is not readily available from the manufacturers. This makes it difficult for clinicians or consumers to estimate fluoride ingestion from carbonated beverages. (Heilman)

Aspertame, another dangerous chemical found in soda pop (and in many "diet" foods), has been linked to numerous health problems including migraine headaches, prostate cancer, memory loss, seizures, obesity, pain, infertility, etc. The official FDA list contains a total of 92 health complaints from thousands and thousands of people associated with this artificial sweetener.

Coke: The Real Thing

To clean a toilet: *Pour a can of Coca-Cola into the toilet bowl. Let the "real thing" sit for one hour, then flush clean. The acid in Coke removes stains from vitreous china.*

To remove rust spots from chrome car bumpers: *Rub the bumper with a crumpled up piece of aluminum foil dipped in Coca-Cola.*

To clean corrosion from car battery terminals: *Pour a can of Coca-Cola over the terminals to bubble away corrosion.*

To loosen a rusted bolt: *Apply a cloth soaked in Coca-Cola to the rusted bolt for several minutes.*

To bake a moist ham: *Empty a can of Coca-Cola into the baking pan. Wrap the ham in aluminum foil and bake. 30 minutes before the ham is finished, remove the foil allowing the drippings to mix with the Coke for a brown gravy.*

To remove grease from clothes: *Empty a can of Coke into a load of greasy clothes, add detergent, and run through a regular wash cycle.*

Coca-Cola will help loosen grease stains. It will also clean road haze from your windshield.

The active ingredient in Coke is phosphoric acid. It's pH is 2.8. It will dissolve a nail in about 4 days.

To carry Coca-Cola syrup (the concentrate), a commercial truck must use the HazMat (Hazardous material) placecards reserved for highly corrosive materials.

The distributors of Coke have been using it to clean the engines of their truck for about 20 years.

The Sin of Caffeine, Alcohol & other Chemicals

It is difficult for many people to understand what is so bad about drinking coffee and other caffeinated beverages, sweets, soda pop, alcohol, cigarettes, etc.

Ask yourself, "*if I eat or drink this, is it bringing glory to God?*" (1 Corinthians 10:31) Or do you want it because it will bring glory to you (and your fleshly desires)?

For example, I am not saying that having a cup of coffee is a sin. However, it is a good idea to take a look at your attitude towards these things. Have you ever said anything like, "I haven't had my coffee yet" or "Gotta have my coffee." Would you make a special trip to the store just because you were out of coffee (or cigarettes, soda pop, etc.)?

Carol said:

> I knew that God was telling me to cut back on my coffee intake. I usually drank coffee at work, but during one particularly stressful period, I started drinking more than my usual one cup. I found myself making a pot of coffee on the weekends, which I had never done in the past because my husband did not drink coffee. I even started drinking caffeinated beverages. At the same time I had developed a very painful lump in the back of my neck that was causing horrible headaches. God was really putting it on my heart that it was due to my caffeine

intake. I finally listened to Him and stopped drinking coffee and caffeine all together. After one week, the headaches were gone and the lump was almost gone too. I think it's really about listening to God and obedience.

It is not necessarily the food – it is often how much we eat of it or how much importance we give to it. If it makes you nervous to give it up – if you think it would be a sacrifice – then it is something you perhaps should think about doing.

This goes for food, supplements, alcohol, drugs, cigarettes, and many other things:

This pill will help me lose weight.

This pill will give me energy.

This pill will calm my stomach because I ate too much.

This pill will numb my pain.

This pill will help me sleep.

This pill will calm me down.

This drink will help me reduce stress.

You get the picture.

Caffeine

Americans consume nearly 500 million cups of coffee each day. The average person drinks 25 gallons a year. Caffeine is the most widely consumed drug in Western society. In addition to coffee, caffeine is also found in tea, chocolate, weight-loss products, pain relievers and cold remedies.

Ninety-nine percent of ingested caffeine is absorbed and distributed to all tissues and organs. The effects of caffeine intake differ greatly according to acute or chronic intake, level of intake and the development of tolerance. Caffeine administered to non-users or recent abstainers can induce hypertension, arrhythmias, altered myocardial function, increased plasma catecholamine levels, plasma renin activity, serum cholesterol levels, increased production of urine, gastric acid secretion and alterations in mood and sleep patterns. Tolerance to chronic caffeine intake develops in most individuals, with the cessation of its effects on the kidneys, the cardiovascular system, the gastrointestinal system and, to some extent, the central nervous system. (Leonard)

Studies clearly show that caffeine increases blood pressure and has an even stronger effect in hypertensive individuals. Most researchers conclude that regular coffee may be harmful to some hypertension-prone subjects. (Nurminen)

With age, the body (particularly your brain) becomes more sensitive to caffeine, so you are more susceptible to many of its adverse effects, including tremors, insomnia, anxiety, panic attacks, irritability, rapid heartbeat, muscle twitching and abdominal pain.

The amount of caffeine it takes to trigger these side effects varies from person to person, but many researchers suspect that as little as 300 mg. (about three six-ounce cups of coffee) may be too much for some people.

Coffee and Heart Disease

Studies show that people who drank more than five cups of coffee per day are 60% more likely to develop heart disease and an increased risk of death from heart disease. There's also a correlation between a high coffee intake and high levels of total cholesterol and LDL cholesterol. When people with elevated cholesterol stop drinking coffee, their cholesterol drops by about 10%.

Drinkers of boiled coffee have higher cholesterol levels than drinkers of filtered coffee. The filters may help remove cholesterol-raising culprits.

Moderation Is The Key

A low intake, 100 to 200 mgs. of caffeine (1-2 cups of drip coffee a day, or two shots of espresso) has no proven link to disease. With higher intakes, 500 mgs. of caffeine or four or more cups of coffee a day (depending on the strength), there is no question of increased risk of many serious diseases.

Some people should avoid coffee and caffeine all together. You should abstain if you have a heart rhythm disorder, high blood pressure, panic disorder, fibrocystic breast disease, or if you are a pregnant woman or trying to become pregnant.

If you drink more than two cups of coffee a day, you are probably addicted to caffeine. You should cut back until you can enjoy just an occasional cup. If you abruptly stop drinking coffee it may cause severe headaches, fatigue and depression, so you're better off gradually tapering your consumption.

If you are thinking of switching to decaf, you may

want to reconsider. When coffee is decaffeinated, some of the chemicals used to extract the caffeine are left behind, creating other health problems, especially in the liver. Trichloroethylene is a particularly nasty cancer-causing agent (the FDA allows up to 10 parts per million in instant coffee and 25 parts per million in ground, roasted decaffeinated coffee). Other commonly used chemicals — trichloroethane, ethyl acetate, and methylene chloride — are also potent carcinogens. If you really want to drink decaf, drink only water-extracted decaf.

Alcohol

Alcohol, like caffeine is a diuretic, which increases the need for water as it increases water loss through the urinary system. Also flushed out, are many water-soluble nutrients.

The federal Office of Technology Assessment estimates that alcoholism and alcohol abuse cost the United States up to $120 billion annually in lost productivity, law enforcement, property damage, health care and alcoholism treatment programs. This sum doesn't reflect the immeasurable losses from human pain and suffering. More than 100,000 deaths per year are directly attributable to alcohol. After cigarettes, alcohol is the second most avoidable cause of death in the United States.

The following are a few of the health problems associated with alcohol use and abuse:

Anger/Aggression	Anxiety
Cancer	Fatigue
Depression	Headaches
Hearing & Sight Problems	Heart Disease
Immune System Depression	Liver Damage
Malnutrition	Memory Loss
Neurological Effects	Osteoporosis
Pancreatitis	Diabetes
Sexual Problems	Sleep Disorders
Stomach Ulceration	Stress/Irritability
Birth Defects	Candida Yeast
Infections	Varicose Veins

Capillary Fragility, Bruising, Spiders, Rosacca, etc.

There are many scriptures which discuss wine and drinking. It does not necessarily say that wine is forbidden, but strongly encourages responsible use:

Wine is a mocker, strong drink is raging: and whosoever is deceived thereby is not wise. Proverbs 20:1

He that loveth pleasure shall be a poor man: he that loveth wine and oil shall not be rich. Proverbs 21:17

And be not drunk with wine, wherein is excess; but be filled with the Spirit. Ephesians 5:18

Not given to wine, no striker, not greedy of filthy lucre; but patient, not a brawler, not covetous. 1Timothy 3:3

The aged women likewise, that they be in behavior as becometh holiness, not false accusers, not given to much wine, teachers of good things. Titus 2:3

There are certain times where scripture states it may be appropriate to drink wine such as in celebration or in mourning: *And wine that maketh glad the heart of man, and oil to make his face to shine, and bread which strengtheneth man's heart* (Psalms 104:15). *Give strong drink unto him that is ready to perish, and wine unto those that be of heavy hearts* (Proverbs 31:6). However, *It is not for kings, O Lemuel, it is not for kings to drink wine; nor for princes strong drink:* Proverbs 31:4. This clearly tells us that if you have certain responsibilities (including driving a vehicle), it is not the time to be drinking wine or other stronger drinks.

It is also inappropriate to drink if it causes someone else to stumble: *It is good neither to eat flesh, nor to drink wine, nor any thing whereby thy brother stumbleth, or is offended, or is made weak.* Romans 14:21

Wine for Health

Drink no longer water, but use a little wine for thy stomach's sake and thine often infirmities. 1Timothy 5:23

In this section of Paul's letter to Timothy, he encourages him to take care of his health. Paul advises him to use wine for the helping of his stomach and the recruiting of his nature. Obviously *a little wine* is important as we must not be given *to much* wine, which would hamper one's health.

Matthew Henry writes: *God has made wine to rejoice man's heart. It is the will of God that people should take all due care of their bodies. As we are not to make them our masters, so neither our slaves; but to use them so that they may be most fit and helpful to us in the service of God... Wine should be used as a help, and not a hindrance, to our health and usefulness.*

As you may know, red wine does contain powerful health promoting components: polyphenols and anthocyanes. Researchers have shown a number of their health promoting effects, including support of the cardiovascular system. In *moderate* consumption, wine can reduce mortality from coronary heart disease by increasing HDL cholesterol (the good one) and inhibiting platelet aggregation and it can also have a favorable effect on triglyceride levels. (Ardevol)

In countries where wine is the primary alcoholic drink, heart disease death rates are lowest. Interestingly, the opposite is true for beer. Where higher amounts of beer are consumed (like in the US), heart disease rates are higher, Red wine, in the amount of <u>one glass</u> per day, seems to elevate HDL, the "good" cholesterol, which helps protect us against heart disease.

The many antioxidant phytochemicals such as polyphenols and flavonoids in red wine have a variety of specific health benefits: They promote nitric oxide production, inhibit platelet aggregation (clotting), help regulate cholesterol levels, and arrest tumor growth to protect us against cancer. (Soleas)

Polyphenols in wine, in addition to their antioxidant effects, are also antimicrobial. They are effective against cholera, the dreaded E. coli, and also E. typhi. The Greeks and others used to pour wine into wounds and over dressings to disinfect them. (Soleas)

Very importantly, the Bible strongly encourages us to not allow wine and alcohol (by consuming too much) to confuse our minds and judgement.

Who has woe? Who has sorrow? Who has strife? Who has complaints? Who has needless bruises? Who has bloodshot eyes? Those who linger over wine, who go to sample bowls of mixed wine. Do not gaze at wine when it is red, when it sparkles in the cup, when it goes down smoothly! In the end it bites like a snake and poisons like a viper. Your eyes will see strange sights and your mind imagine confusing things. You will be like one sleeping on the high seas, lying on top of the rigging. "They hit me," you will say, "but I'm not hurt! They beat me, but I don't feel it! When will I wake up so I can find another drink?" Proverbs 23:29-35

Be sober, be vigilant; because your adversary the devil, as a roaring lion, walketh about, seeking whom he may devour. 1Peter 5:8

Satan will use any way he can to get his way. Too much alcohol (which may be very little for some people) can cause one to lose self control. Too much wine makes you foolish, opening the door of opportunity for Satan to take advantage of you, in your weakened state. Many people will do and say things they never would if they were not under the influence. This is what God wants to prevent. It is for our own protection that we do not abuse alcohol. If we do, there are likely to be consequences. Some people have lost everything they have because of their love for alcohol. Alcohol is a drug and can become addictive when abused.

For the grace of God that bringeth salvation hath appeared to all men, Teaching us that, denying ungodliness and worldly lusts, we should live soberly, righteously, and godly, in this present world. Titus 2:11-12

Other Chemicals

While God entrusted man with the care of his perfect creation, there are 600 to even 1,000 man-made carcinogenic (cancer-causing) chemicals now polluting and poisoning our food, water and environment. These toxic chemicals are difficult for both the earth and our bodies to handle. We do not have enzymes to metabolize these chemcials as it was obviously not God's desire that we pollute his creation.

As a consequence, our health, and the state of earth have greatly suffered. Cancer rates are currently as high as one out of every two people in some parts of the United States. Ninety percent of all cancers are related to environmental exposure – cigarette smoke, pesticides and other such chemicals, high fat, low fiber diet, etc.

Western medicine is largely responsible for our environmental pollution. This is the "magic bullet," "attack and conquer" approach — kill the germs, spray the bugs, add more chemicals to the soil to stimulate growth. If things get worse or side effects develop, use a different or stronger chemical. It is an endless cycle because this approach is continually reaching for a new series of effects rather than addressing the causes. The problem will never be corrected this way. There will always be germs and insects. Spraying to kill them and those pesky weeds, may seem to yield a better crop and more profits – but at what expense to our health down the road?

When the concentration of chemicals used in our food chain, at home, or in industry rises to a certain level, there are side effects – everything from mild irritations to blood and immunological disorders. Our body may be stressed by chemical insults, whether we breathe them, drink them or eat them. This stress increases our potential for disease as it stresses the immune system. Many radiation and air-borne chemicals are well-known causes of many specific diseases and cancers. Often, however, we do not find out that these chemicals are dangerous to humans until they have been in use for years.

The health of the environment and the health of our bodies are closely aligned. If the environment is sick, we cannot be healthy. Pollution in many forms occurs alone, upon, and within our planet and in every person's body.

We are bombarded with an abundance of environmental pseudo-estrogens or xenoestrogens (*xeno* means "foreign," so *xenoestrogens* means "foreign estrogens") in western civilized societies, creating an imbalance with our other hormones, primarily progesterone.

Estrogen replacement therapy (unopposed estrogen without progesterone), hysterectomy, birth control pills, exposure to xenoestrogens and dietary abundance all contribute to estrogen dominance. Excess calories with an abundance of animal fats, sugars, refined starches and processed foods lead to estrogen levels in women that are twice as high as women in third-world countries. This sets the stage for an exaggerated estrogen decline at menopause. (Lee)

Problems associated with estrogen dominance:

Pre and post menopausal bone loss

Allergies	Diminished sex drive
Depression	Fatigue
Fibrocystic breasts	Increased blood clotting

Infertility (in men and women)

Miscarriage	PMS
Uterine cancer	Uterine fibroids

Water retention

Fat gain (especially around the belly, hips, thighs)

Xenoestrogens are known to cause:

Infertility   Premature puberty

Fibrocystic breast disease   Breast cancer

PMS *and who knows what else!*

Note: Do not confuse xenoestrogens with phyto-estrogens which are naturally found in soy and many other plants and herbs (black cohosh, damiana, dong quai, wild yam, etc.). These are found to be protective against the above health problems.

Environmental pollutants play a key role in many of our current health problems, including breast cancer (now at epidemic levels), PMS, infertility and fibrocystic breast disease. Xenoestrogens are found in everyday synthetic materials — materials which were previously thought to be inert. They include: DDT (the pesticide), PCBs (industrial chemicals known as polychlorinated biphenyls) and DDE (a DDT breakdown product).

The use of DDT has been banned in the United States since 1972 because of its harm to our health and environment – it does not breakdown, it just remains in the soil. In the body, DDT and DDE are stored in the fat cells and continue to poison the body for many years. It is still not known for how long after one is exposed.

In the year 2000, a worldwide ban of the manufacture of DDT became effective, but it will take another four to seven years before the current supplies are expected to be depleted as it is sold to other countries. We, in the United States, then purchase their produce and crops which were sprayed with it.

According the the Agency for Toxic Substances and Disease Registry, in a Public Health Statement, small amounts of DDT and DDE can still be found in soil and water and even some crops grown today in areas where the chemical was used prior to the ban.

The body's hormones are at levels of parts per trillion. However, these chemicals that affect the sex-hormone systems of the human body occur at 100 to 1,000 times greater concentration than that of normal human hormones. To function in optimal health – including optimal sexual health, the sex hormones, including estrogen, progesterone, testosterone, DHEA, etc., all need to be at their proper level and in balance with each other. If not, problems occur.

Exposure to pesticides and other pollutants having estrogenic effects for an extended period results in feminization, including a lower sperm count and breast development in men, early puberty and premenstrual (PMS) problems in women.

Feminization is taking place: In Lake Opopka, Florida, there was a big spill of an estrogenic pesticide in 1988. Subsequently, male alligators developed abnormally small reproductive organs, reproductive impairment and female-like hormone levels. Florida panthers were exposed to the estrogenic pesticide DDT for years, and they ate other animals that were also exposed. They found that the panther fatty tissue had high levels of DDE, a DDT breakdown product. They had low sperm counts, unusually high levels of abnormal sperm, undescended testicles and thyroid dysfunction.

In the lower Columbia River in the Northwest, juvenile male otters have testicles that are only one-seventh normal weight. They, too, show evidence of exposure to estrogenic chemicals.

This is another reason why eating organically raised foods is so important. Unfortunately, they usually cost more, so if you cannot grow your own, this is the risk you take. Recommendations:

- Use simple soaps and detergents with less chemicals.

- Use natural pest control not pesticides.

- Avoid synthetic chemicals.

- Do not use herbicides.

- Eat only hormone-free meats.

- Eat only organic food grown without pesticides, herbicides or synthetic fertilizers or hormones.

- Avoid spermicides and birth control pills for birth control.

- Phytoestrogens found in soy (and soy products tempeh, tofu, etc.), black cohosh, damiana, dong quai, wild yam, chaste berry, etc. can be helpful to help balance estrogen, progesterone and other sex hormones.

- The botanical extract tribulus terrestris is helpful for men and women to restore normal testosterone levels and reproductive functioning without side effects.

Nutrition

Nutrition is the relationship between foods and the health of the body. Optimal nutrition is a diet that contains all essential nutrients that are supplied and utilized in a balanced amount to maintain good health.

But, in order for the body to do this, it must be properly nourished. The body is not indestructible. Natural aging, environmental stresses and some genetic factors do play a role, but proper nutrition is by far the largest factor in our ability to maintain optimal health.

Knowledge of the nutrients and their functions in the body is helpful for achieving good nutrition and a balanced diet. A balanced diet contains portions of each of the six main nutrient classifications of food: carbohydrates, proteins, fats, vitamins, minerals and water.

Each nutrient has its own special function and relationship to the body, but no nutrient acts independently of the other. All the nutrients must be present in the right quantities in order to maintain optimum health. Although everyone requires all these nutrients, individuals do not necessarily require the same amounts. Quantities vary according to individual needs.

In spite of all the excuses we might have for not getting proper nutrients such as soil depletion, food processing and cooking, it ultimately is our own responsibility to feed ourselves properly. Too often, we sacrifice optimal nutrition for convenience, cost or taste.

As a nation of convenience, we want what is fast

and easy. We have a huge abundance of fast food restaurants, frozen foods, canned foods, boxed foods and junk foods to choose from to satisfy our hunger and cravings. Unfortunately, refining processes and the preservatives and additives that accompany them are preventing us from satisfying our nutritional needs.

Many people mistakenly believe that the typical American diet is well-balanced and contains sufficient amounts of all the nutrients we need for optimum health. However, North American surveys show that the diets of more than 60% of the people tested are deficient in one or more of the essential nutrients. Most surveys test only 10 of the 45 known nutrients and use the standard Daily Value (DV) System, which is considered very low. Recognized as the minimal requirements for survival, DVs are inadequate to maintain optimum health.

The most common deficiencies found in these surveys were iron, calcium, zinc, chromium, potassium, iodine, magnesium, selenium, manganese, Vitamins C, A, E, B-6, B-2, folic acid, essential fatty acids (Omega-3 and Omega-6) and antioxidants.

Nutritional deficiencies result whenever tissues are deprived of adequate amounts of essential nutrients over a long period of time. Good nutrition is essential for: normal organ development and functioning, nor-

Use your food as your medicine and your medicine as your food. Hippocrates

mal reproduction and growth, optimal energy and efficiency, resistance to infection and disease, and the repair of bodily damage or injuries.

Deficiency symptoms are not necessarily obvious. Conditions develop slowly over time and can be very insidious and difficult to identify. One does not need to have scurvy to have a Vitamin C deficiency. One does not need to have osteoporosis to have a calcium deficiency. Symptoms can be as subtle as appetite loss, bad breath, soft or brittle fingernails, fatigue or insomnia.

We are not exactly healthy as a population. We suffer from fatigue, frequent colds, allergies, excessive weight, diabetes, hypoglycemia, anemia, arthritis, mental problems, heart disease, cancer and many other conditions that leave us unsatisfied with our health and feeling poorly. We too often do not even consider our own eating habits as the possible cause.

This information is important. You need to know how important these things are to obtain and maintain good health.

Epidemiological studies indicate that a diet rich in fruits and vegetables may lower the incidence of cancer and other degenerative conditions. This preventive effect could be due to the numerous benefits that these foods provide us with. They are low in calories, low in fat, and supply us with various vitamins, minerals, antioxidants and phytochemicals – specific medicinal compounds derived from plants. (Hocman)

Researchers are now just starting to understand how the hundreds of different phytonutrients in fruits and vegetables and whole grains enhance our immune

> A Harvard study recently published in the *American Journal of Clinical Nutrition* suggests that a higher intake of fruit and vegetables is protective against cardiovascular disease and diabetes supporting the theory to increase fruit and vegetable intake. (Liu)

systems and prevents disease. The mechanisms of prevention include enhanced enzymatic detoxification of harmful compounds, and inhibition of their binding to cellular DNA, their fiber content, detoxification of radical forms of carcinogens by their natural antioxidants and probably many other ways too.

Free radicals play a critical role in the development of the two diseases responsible for two out of every three deaths. The Mayo Clinic reports that approximately 43% of deaths in the United States are due to some form of cardiovascular disease and 23% are caused by cancer.

Almost 10 years ago, the Surgeon General's Report on Nutrition and Health stated that making the correct dietary choices could decrease our cancer risk by 35 - 60%. The National Cancer Institute (NCI) even opened a Cancer Research Laboratory devoted solely to investigating the role of diet in cancer prevention and treatment. Numerous studies have already demonstrated the protective relationship between fruit and vegetable intake and cancers of the lung, colon, breast, cervix, esophagus, mouth and throat, stomach, bladder, pancreas and ovary.

While the U.S. Surgeon General recommends five to nine servings of fruits and vegetables daily, the *Journal of Nutrition* reports that just one out of 10 Americans eats even five servings. The best way to eat fruits and vegetable is raw or cooked (better than canned), preferably lightly steamed and not microwaved, which can destroy their delicate balance of anticarcinogenic ingredients.

Another large Harvard study, conducted over eight years, identified two major dietary patterns for the development of coronary artery disease. The "low risk factor" was characterized by higher intake of vegetables, fruits, legumes, whole grains, fish, and poultry, whereas the "high risk factor," also called the "Western pattern," was characterized by higher intake of red meat, processed meat, refined grains, sweets and dessert, French fries, and high-fat dairy products. (Hu)

So why don't we eat our fruits and veggies?

1. It's difficult to get to the market everyday to purchase a fresh supply.

2. Time required for preparation.

3. Expense. (What ever happened to gardening?)

4. Pesticides and other chemicals contaminate our produce making it extremely difficult to find 100% pure fruits and vegetables. Even certified organically grown produce may contain up to 10% pesticide residues.

5. And last, but not least, not everyone likes the

taste of certain foods just because they are good for us. It is important to introduce a variety of fruits and vegetables to children so they become accustomed to their taste.

Areas Recommended for Improvement for Most People:

1. **Increase intake of essential fatty acids, especially Omega-3.**

2. **Increase intake of fiber.**

3. **Increase intake of fruits, vegetables and other whole foods.** (For adequate intake of anti-oxidants, phytochemicals and other important nutrients found in these foods.)

1. Essential Fatty Acids (EFAs)

Not all fat is bad. The fact is, we need some fat in our diet, but we need the *right kind*. Of the 45 essential nutrients that must be obtained from foods, two are fatty acids: Omega-6 (linoleic acid), a polyunsaturated EFA, and Omega-3 (alpha-linolenic acid), a super-unsaturated EFA. Arachidonic acid is considered essential, but it can be synthesized in the body if sufficient linoleic and linolenic are present. The reason they are called *essential* is the body cannot manufacture them and they must be ingested daily.

Essential fatty acids are necessary for normal growth and healthy blood arteries and nerves. Essential fatty acids are important for the transport and breakdown of cholesterol. They also keep skin and other tissues youthful and healthy. Essential fatty acids are the highest source of energy in nutrition.

Omega-3 is vital to brain development, normal blood pressure, healthy skin and an effective immune system. They also lower triglycerides and cholesterol, if levels are elevated. The anti-aggregatory, anti-thrombotic and anti-inflammatory properties of Omega-3 have all been clinically demonstrated.

Omega-3 oils are broken down into two active substances, EPA (eicosapentaenoic acid) and DHA (docohexaenoic acid). EPA has been specifically shown to play an important role in heart health. DHA is very important for proper brain growth and development.

The two major sources of Omega-3 are **cold water fish** and **flax seeds** – two foods many people rarely eat.

Flaxseed oil requires less processing than fish oils, can be produced without pollutants, breaks down less readily, and is more cost effective to produce commercially. Flax is also higher in Omega-3 than fish.

Excellent fish sources include:

Salmon, trout, tuna, anchovies, mackerel, haddock and herring.

Small amounts can also be found in:

Soybeans and **soybean oil**

Sunflower, sesame and **pumpkin seeds** and **oil**

Walnuts

Garbanzo beans (chick peas)

Dark green vegetables, such as fresh broccoli and **spinach**

To obtain essential fatty acids in the diet, it is best to rely upon fresh, raw, unrefined foods or products like fresh, unrefined cold-pressed oils.

Omega-3 and Omega-6 fatty acids are essential to good health. These two EFAs form the membranes of every one of the billions of cells in our bodies. They are also needed for cellular energy production. Glands need EFAs to carry out the secretion of hormones and other regulating substances. Muscles require EFAs to repair damaged tissues and to speed healing. EFAs are critical to the immune response. Brain, eye, adrenal and nerve cells require EFAs to function, and EFAs are necessary for growth and reproduction. Additionally, EFAs are converted into prostaglandins.

Omega-3 and Omega-6 are prostaglandin precursors (or raw materials). Prostaglandins are key body substances that regulate nearly every physical function. Prostaglandins support or control the following:

- Inflammation

- Healing and repair

- Immune system

- Neural circuits in the brain

- Cardiovascular system including cholesterol levels and actions in the bloodstream

- Blood pressure

- Blood coagulation (helps keep platelets from sticking together – clots)

- Digestive and reproductive systems

- Body thermostat and calorie burning

- Cell growth and proliferation

As we age, our bodies become less efficient at the process of converting Omega-3 into these helpful prostaglandins. Several diseases, including cancer, eczema, multiple sclerosis and diabetes, also make the conversion less efficient.

How Much?

It is not only important to consume adequate amounts of Omega-3 and Omega-6 fatty acids, it is also very important to consume them in the proper ratio. An excessive intake of Omega-6 is much easier to obtain in the diet because it is found in corn, safflower and other commonly-consumed vegetable oils.

In recent years, the incidence of asthma and allergies has increased. There is an interesting correlation with the recent change of our dietary fat consumption. There is a reduced intake of saturated (animal) fats, an increase in the intake of polyunsaturated fatty acids from vegetable oils containing Omega-6, and a *decrease* in the intake of oily fish which contains Omega-3.

Omega-6 is the precursor to *inflammatory* prostaglandins. Omega-3 *inhibits prostaglandin E2,* thereby, helping to regulate our inflammatory response. (Black, Wenzel) It is easy to see how our anti-inflammatory response may be inhibited by a diet lacking in fish, flax or other sources of Omega-3.

Fats to Avoid

There is absolutely no biological need in the body body for saturated fat - fats that are solid at room temperature. The liver can manufacture all the cholesterol the body needs if adequate unsaturated fatty acids are available. Saturated fats are   animal products such as dairy (cheese, cream, etc.), meat and eggs.

Hydrogenated and partially hydrogenated fats are fats that have been changed from their natural liquid form to become more solid (like saturated fats). These altered fats should be avoided because this processing changes the natural molecular structure of the fatty acids into an unnatural trans-configuration. These trans-fatty acids are unhealthy because they resemble saturated fats but the body has a much more difficult time processing them. Trans-fatty acids also produce free radicals in the body. Because very few amounts of trans-fatty acids occur in nature, they are *foreign* to the body.

Hydrogenated fats are saturated-like fats made from plant oils and fats that have been heated to very high temperatures (as high as 458°) and pressure-processed. Enzymes are killed at much lower temperatures, therefore all active enzymes are eliminated.

Hydrogenated fats are created when an oil that is largely unsaturated, such as corn oil, has hydrogen added to it, causing fat to become more solid at room temperature.

During hydrogenation, the unsaturated fat becomes more saturated. Hydrogenated oils are *artificially saturated* fats. The more solid and hydrogenated the fat, the more trans-fatty acids there are in the product. Examples of hydrogenated fat products include margarine, margarine-based products, shortenings, and fats used for frying.

Don't ever believe anyone who tries to tell you that margarine is healthier than butter. **Butter is natural -** the body knows how to process it (in moderation), Margarine is full of trans-fatty acids just waiting to get hung up in your arteries. (Valenzuela) JUST SAY NO TO MARGARINE and ALTERED FATS!

Note: Almost all processed foods contain altered fats. Check food labels for <u>hydrogenated</u> or <u>partially hydrogenated</u> oils – and then put if back on the shelf.

Why are Trans-fatty Acids Bad?

Among other results, researchers have found that trans-fatty acids significantly raise LDL cholesterol levels, the bad cholesterol, while lowering the HDL levels, the good cholesterol – even more so than saturated fats. (Valenzuela) In the Framingham Heart Study (a 40-year study covering 5,209 individuals living in Massachusetts) high LDL cholesterol levels combined with low HDL levels were indicative of increased coronary heart disease risk.

These trans-fatty acids can easily become trapped along arterial walls creating an ideal environment for build-up of plaque and development of atherosclerosis.

Results from other human studies and recent large-scale epidemiologic surveys also clearly show that dietary trans-fatty acids enhance the risk of developing coronary heart diseases. Studies support the idea that lowering current intakes of trans-fatty acids may lower the risk of coronary heart disease. (Nelson GJ)

Other healthier fats are the monounsaturated fats found in avocados, olives and olive oil.

2. Fiber

Fiber plays a major role in maintaining a healthy digestive tract. The term fiber refers to or encompasses several carbohydrates and lignans that resist breakdown by human digestive enzymes and that are fermented by the microflora of the colon.

Soluble fiber such as in oat bran, wheat bran, psyllium and apple and fruit pectin provides the following health benefits:

- Absorbs toxins for elimination from the body

- Provides food for beneficial bacteria in the colon

- Controls blood sugar levels by slowing down blood sugar absorption

- Improves cholesterol levels in the blood by lowering the bad LDL and raising the good HDL

- Reduces heart disease risk

- Reduces colon cancer risk

Insoluble fiber such as lignan, cellulose, and chitosan is barely fermentable and provides the following health benefits:

- Provides a laxative and intestinal regulatory effect

- Acts like a broom to sweep the intestines clean

- Regulates bowel activity (constipation and diarrhea)

- Aids digestion

- Reduces colon cancer risk

In the colon, fiber holds onto water, which helps form a softer, larger, more consistent bowel movement. Fiber also carries bile and fat out of the body. Without fiber, much of this fat is reabsorbed and recirculated.

By helping cleanse fat and debris (toxins) from the digestive tract, nitrogen and sulphur gasses are also reduced, allowing for more optimal absorption of important nutrients, including oxygen, which increases the metabolic rate in the body and is important for memory and energy levels.

Fiber is an excellent weight loss aid as it helps eliminate excess dietary fat through the digestive tract that would otherwise contribute to weight gain and formation of excess gasses.

Effect of Fiber on Insulin

When you a eat a high carbohydrate food without its natural fiber, too much sugar is too quickly dumped into your blood stream, causing production of too much insulin. The job of insulin is to "take" the glucose into the cells to be burned for energy. Too much insulin initiates an enzyme to tell our brain that there is too much glucose, and the ability of the liver to store any excess is exceeded. The remaining glucose is stored as fat.

Fiber slows the breakdown of carbohydrates in the stomach. Removing fiber (for example, when you squeeze an orange to produce orange juice), allows the carbohydrates to rapidly convert into simple sugars and to quickly enter the bloodstream.

Lack of fiber is associated with:

Cardiovascular disease	*Colon cancer*
Gallstones	*Ulcerative colitis*
Diverticulitis	*Hemorrhoids*
Constipation	*Skin problems*

It is far better to eat the whole orange, than just to drink the juice and throw away the fiber. Notice how much fuller you feel after eating a whole apple compared to drinking a glass of apple juice.

Fiber Content in Foods: Highest to Lowest

1. **Whole grain cereals** – whole grain wheat, corn, barley, rye, buckwheat, millet, oats, rice, amaranth and flax

2. **Legumes** – peas, beans, lentils
    Nuts
    Seeds
    Dried fruits

3. **Root vegetables** – potatoes, yams, kohlrabi, carrots, parsnips, turnips, beets

4. **Fruits**
    Leafy vegetables – lettuce, cabbage, celery

5. **Animal products** contain **NO FIBER**
    Beef, pork, chicken, fish and other meats, eggs, milk and milk products (cheese, yogurt, etc.)

Benefits of a High Fiber Diet

The health benefits of a high-fiber diet are practically too numerous to list. Fiber is simply a necessary dietary component which really went unnoticed until we started suffering the effects of eating a diet without it.

One particular study on fiber in the treatment of obesity and elevated cholesterol demonstrated how the daily addition of just 15 grams (2 teaspoons) of a high fiber food supplement could result in a significant weight loss and also a drop in blood cholesterol levels. (Kaul)

Fiber is a very important component of food and one of the main reasons foods should be eaten in their whole, natural form (the way God created it). Some of the health benefits of fiber include the following:

Fiber Benefits:

- Helps you feel full and eat less.

- Holds water and increases fecal bulk.

- Binds bile acids carrying them (and fats) out of the body.

- Reduces or normalizes transit time.

- Causes fermentation in the large bowel (it provides something for the bacteria to grow upon).

- Helps fight constipation and bloating.

- Lowers the risk of colon-rectal cancer – the second leading cause of death in this country.

- Improves colon health by "keeping things moving." Benefits symptoms of irritable bowel.

- Speeds elimination of toxins and waste products.

- Reduces elevated cholesterol.

- Lowers risk of heart disease – the leading cause of death in this country.

Transit Time

Transit time is the period it takes for food to travel from the mouth until it exits the body as waste. Because of the inadequate fiber in the diets of so many people, transit time is too slow in most people. The slower the transit time, the longer toxic waste remains in the body. This allows more time for putrification to occur amongst the waste materials. This can lead to production of unhealthy waste products – including carcinogenic substances. These residues can even be reabsorbed into the blood stream causing metabolic disruptions, skin problems and other complications.

You can check your digestive transit time yourself. Swallow a few kernels of whole corn without chewing. Transit time varies with the food you consume, so continue to eat the foods you normally do. Watch to see how long it takes for the corn to appear in your stool. A healthy normal range would be between 12-18 hours.

If it takes less than 10 hours, there may not have been adequate time for proper digestion and assimilation of the nutrients in your food. The exception to this would be if you are already consuming a very high fiber diet and the stools are well formed, not loose.

If it takes longer than 24 hours, you can consider yourself constipated and it would be very wise to consume more fiber and drink more water. Variation of transit time can range from 47 to 123 hours in the same person, depending on diet, drug and fluid intake.

A wonderful thing about fiber is that it helps normalize the digestive tract whether it is working too slow or too fast.

A Country of Constipated People

Did you know that the average transit time for young healthy adults in Western countries is an unbelievable three days? In Third World countries, the average transit time is less than 18 hours. You don't see colon cancer in these countries. In the United States, constipation is a huge problem - which is also further reflected in our high incidence of colon cancer. Colon cancer is the second most common form of cancer. Among the elderly, some individuals do not pass a bowel movement for as many as 14 days.

Constipation is not only uncomfortable, it is very unhealthy. Toxins from fermenting waste products can be reabsorbed into the blood stream, creating all sorts of problems ranging from fatigue and skin problems to colon cancer. Bacteria react with bile salts to form carcinogens.

In addition to fiber, there are many cleansing foods (especially those high in chlorophyll which provides a dark green color) which help remove toxins from the body. These include alfalfa, spinach, romaine lettuce, brocoli and other green vegetable. Algea, such as spirulina and chorella, are also high in chlorophyll.

It is far better to consume natural whole foods (complete with fiber and other nutrients) as our Creator made them rather than isolated from its natural source and taken alone, such as psyllium husks, or the bran of grains. Oat bran is beneficial, but it is better to eat the whole oat, not just the bran.

3. Whole Foods

God has a plan for everything. The whole basis behind nature is for everything to work together, nothing in isolation, to use everything to its full potential, wasting nothing.

In nature, nothing exists in isolation. You won't find ascorbic acid or magnesium growing on a tree somewhere. It is best to use foods (whenever possible) as God intended in their natural, whole form.

A more natural diet satisfies hunger because it satisfies the body's need for nutrition – vitamins, minerals, fiber, complex carbohydrates, etc. Processing removes many of these components which the body needs. Sometimes you will see that a refined product is "enriched." It is better to consume natural whole foods which do not need enrichment– as they are perfect as God created them.

● Milk, consumed in it's whole, natural form is very healthy. The milk we buy in the store is processed, and homogenized. The essential fatty acids have been removed and certain nutrients (fat-soluble Vitamins A and D) are lost as a consequence. These are then added back in. Milk today is a far cry from what God intended milk to be.

And I am come down to deliver them out of the hand of the Egyptians, and to bring them up out of that land unto a good land and a large, unto a land flowing with milk and honey. Exodus 3:8

Mass production, commercialization, steroids and antiobiotics have ruined milk and I don't drink it. There are many other excellent sources of calcium to maintain the health of our bones and teeth – spinach, kale, broccoli and other green vegetables, whole grains, nuts, seeds, and beans are all very good sources of *usable* calcium. It is actually hard for the body to assimilate the calcium in milk, in part due to it's high phosphorus content. Milk is also high in protein, which actually increases our need for calcium. Salmon, herring, anchovies, scallops and shrimp also contain usable calcium.

I do love cheese, but cultured cheeses such as feta, cottage cheese and yogurt are easier to digest. I am quite sure yogurt has been around since before Christ.

• Eggs contain fat in the form of cholesterol, but they also contain lecithin to help you emulsify and use the fat. The best way to eat eggs is soft boiled or hard boiled. This way the yolk, which contains the fat, is exposed to the least amount of high heat or oxygen. There are several studies showing that eggs eaten soft boiled do not increase your blood cholesterol level. As with anything, moderation is the key.

• Fruits and vegetables should be eaten whole, not peeled (whenever possible). The peel contains fiber, vitamins, trace minerals, bioflavonoids and many other important trace components, many of which may not even be identified yet. (Buy organic to avoid pesticide residue.)

• Most fruits (and many vegetables) are high in sugar, but the fiber they contain slows down their absorption into the bloodstream preventing too much insulin from being released. It is far better to eat a raw, whole piece of fruit, than to just drink the juice and throw away the fiber.

• Some antioxidants (such as beta carotene) have been shown to be more beneficial when consumed in their whole food form compared to high doses of an isolate in the form of a supplement.

It is well known that fruits and vegetables high in beta carotene offer a protective effect against cancer and some other degenerative diseases. There are many more carotenes and research now shows that they work more effectively in the body together. Beta carotene is just one of dozens of different types of carotenes found in foods. Large amounts of just one form (as in a high potency supplement) can interfere with absorption, transport or use of other forms, causing health problems. (Albanes)

All antioxidants work better in combination with one another. They work together in the body having a synergistic effect.

• Vitamin E also has a number of different naturally occurring forms. It seems that high doses of Alpha-tocopherol may not be such a good idea for cancer protection after all. Because of its cardioprotective effects, a low-dose, mixed tocopherol supplement is advised (200 mg. daily). (Albanes)

A Few of My Favorites

While there are a large number of whole foods with "special" high nutritional value, Here are a few of my "favorites," which I feel are greatly underutilized.

Amaranth

Amaranth, known as the grain of the Aztecs. It is a small seed that resembles millet. It has a mild, nutty flavor. Amaranth can be eaten as a cereal, used in bread, added to soups or salad or eaten as a main dish.

Of all grains, amaranth is the highest in protein content. It is especially rich in lysine, one of the eight essential amino acids, which is usually missing in plant food (but is abundant in animal protein). Amaranth is high in iron and calcium. A two ounce serving of cooked amaranth contains 80% of the DV for iron and 10% of the DV for calcium. Amaranth is also low in fat and calories and high in fiber.

Avocados

These delicious fruits have gotten a bad reputation. Yes, they do contain fat and consequently are high in calories, but they also contain Vitamins A, C and E, niacin, iron, and are very high in B-5, folic acid, potassium and lots of fiber. One medium avocado has as much potassium as three bananas and as much fiber as 42 prunes! Almost all the fat in an avocado is unsaturated and of course, they contain no cholesterol.

Beans and Lentils

Beans and lentils are inexpensive, but hold valuable health benefits. They are an excellent source of protein, yet unlike most other protein sources, have virtually no fat. Lentils, cow peas, black, fava, kidney, lima, pinto, and white beans all contain less than one gram of fat per one-half cup (cooked) serving.

Surprisingly, soy beans contain nine grams of fat per one-half cup (cooked) serving. This fat is largely unsaturated so is still a far better source of protein compared to animal products, which are high in saturated fat.

Beans are mineral-rich too, containing potassium, iron, calcium, magnesium and others.

Did you know that Esau sold Jacob his birthright over a bowl of lentil stew?

And Esau said to Jacob, Feed me, I pray thee, with that same red pottage; for I am faint: therefore was his name called Edom. And Jacob said, Sell me this day thy birthright. And Esau said, Behold, I am at the point to die: and what profit shall this birthright do to me? And Jacob said, Swear to me this day; and he sware unto him: and he sold his birthright unto Jacob. Then Jacob gave Esau bread and pottage of lentiles; and he did eat and drink, and rose up, and went his way: thus Esau despised his birthright. Genesis 25:30-34

Beans come in many different colors, sizes and even shapes, but nutritionally they all have wonderful effects, especially on cholesterol, due to their high content of soluble fiber. Studies show that adding one cup of cooked beans to the daily diet can reduce cholesterol levels by 19%. (Anderson) The insoluble fiber in lentils and beans promotes digestive health.

	Total Fiber
Pinto beans - 1/2 cup	8.8 gms.
Kidney beans - 1/2 cup	7.8 gms.
Lima beans - 1/2 cup	6.4 gms.

Compare to:

Brown rice - 1/2 cup	2 gms.
Whole wheat bread - 1 slice	1.4 gms.
White rice - 1/2 cup	1 gm.

Note: Many people complain that beans give them gas. I have a few suggestions: Eat more of them and chew your food well. Beans are a complex carbohydrate and are difficult to digest. If you do not eat a lot of complex carbohydrate foods, your digestive system may tend to become lazy and sluggish. When you do eat a more challenging food such as beans, your digestive system is not accustomed to working so hard and may not do an adequate job – resulting in partially undigested particles entering the large intestine producing gas.

Chewing is very important because digestion of carbohydrates starts with the digestive enzymes in the mouth. To some extent, the more work you do in the mouth, the less work the rest of the digestive system has to do! CHEW your food well!

Make sure that your beans are cooked well. Also, you may want to start with easier-to-digest legumes such as lentils and peas. Lastly, adding a small amount of baking soda into the water as they cook helps reduce such digestive complaints.

Beets

Beets are amazing. They have incredible health-boosting powers! It's just too bad that they are such a pain in the kitchen to prepare. They have to cook for up to two hours and red dye gets all over everywhere! But, they may be worth it.

Beets are high in both soluble and insoluble fiber. Beet fiber helps to normalize systolic blood pressure, decreases total cholesterol while increasing the beneficial HDL, lowers triglyceride levels, and improves glucose tolerance. Beet fiber also increases absorption of iron and zinc. Just think, all that and **it's not a drug, it's just a vegetable!**

Beets contain iron, which promotes a diuretic washing action through the liver, kidneys and gall bladder. Beets also stimulate movement of lymph fluid, an important component of the immune system.

Beets also contain glutamine, an amino acid which helps keep blood clear of toxins such as ammonia and helps regulate the acid-base balance and electrolytes of the body.

Beets are high in folic acid and Vitamin B-6, but much of it is lost in cooking, so it is best to eat them raw if you can. Juicing in combination with other vegetables is a good way to obtain this benefit.

Cabbage

Cabbage, both green-white and red varieties, is full of valuable health-promoting properties. Very low in calories, cabbage contains almost no sodium or fat, and also contains lots of fiber to cleanse the body of wastes. Red cabbage is high in Vitamin C, sulfur and iron. These minerals cleanse the mucous membranes and wash out fatty deposits acting like a cleansing agent for the stomach and intestinal tract. Cabbage juice is often used to treat and prevent ulcers. Cabbage ranks as one of the best cancer-fighting foods, especially against colon cancer. Some studies indicate that eating cabbage just once a week may cut colon cancer risk by 66%.

Cabbage (and also turnips) contains phenethy isothiocyanate which prevents enzymes from forming carcinogens from potentially harmful substances in our food, drink and also second-hand smoke.

Cabbage (and also soy beans) contains a most remarkable phytochemical, genistein. Genistein prevents the development of capillaries which form around a tumor. Without an adequate supply of oxygen and nutrients, the potential for tumor growth is impeded.

Cabbage also contains cancer-fighting antioxidants that inhibit cholesterol production and provide other protective activities.

The sterols in cabbage are noted for their ability to protect us from breast cancer and block absorption of fats and cholesterol. Other foods containing such sterols include broccoli, cucumbers, yams, sweet potatoes, squash, tomatoes, eggplant, peppers and soy products.

Chili Peppers

Chili peppers, also called cayenne peppers, contain capsaicin, which makes them "hot." Topically, chilis relieve pain, as capsaicin stimulates certain nerve cells to release Substance P, which sends pain signals through-out the nervous system. Capsaicin quickly depletes the cells of Substance P, thus temporarily blocking their ability to transmit pain impulses. Capsaicin ointments are commonly used to alleviate the pain of arthritis and shingles.

Taken internally, capsaicin triggers the release of endorphins in the brain, which has a pain-relieving effect similar to morphine.

Chilis also speed up your metabolism (as much as 25%), which is why after eating hot peppers and foods contain chili seasoning, many people tend to sweat. As a thermogenic, hot peppers may even be an effective weight loss aid. Cayenne stimulates the production of gastric juices and helps relieve gas.

Chilis can also help alleviate the symptoms of the common cold by breaking up congestion and keeping the airways clear. Chili peppers are also rich in beta-carotene (an important antioxidant) and Vitamin C. Chilis may also help lower LDL cholesterol and triglycerides. They also contain antioxidant properties, which help protect against cancer and heart disease. Chili peppers can also prevent blood clots by extending blood coagulation time.

> **Isaiah told the king to put a paste of figs on his boil and he would get well.**
> Isaiah 38:21

Figs

Figs contain benzaldehyde, which provides natural antitumor activity. In one study of 65 patients with inoperable cancer in the advanced stages, 55% of those given benzaldehyde responded favorably; seven patients achieved complete recovery, 29 achieved partial improvement, 24 remained stable, and only five showed progression of the disease. (Kochi) In the Old Testament, Isaiah called for figs to heal King Hezekiah who was "sick unto death" from "a boil," which was probably cancerous. The king recovered.

Figs also contain antibacterial, antiparasitic enzymes called ficins that aid digestion.

Flax Seeds

Flax seeds are an excellent whole food because they are rich in very important nutritional components which are otherwise hard to find. These are the Omega-3 essential fatty acids (linolenic) and lignans, powerful cancer-fighting fibers.

Flax seed, with approximately 60% linolenic acid (LNA), is probably the best source of Omega-3. It also contains the other essential fatty acids, 16% Linoleic

(Omega-6), and 18% Oleic (Omega-9).

Flax seeds are also an excellent source of soluble lignan fiber. Flax seed lignans have a very solid amount of research demonstrating their anti-cancer effects, specifically uterine, cervical and breast cancer. Other research has demonstrated the ability of flax seed lig nans to reduce blood lipids by as much as 27%. (Cunnane)

One serving (20 grams) of flax contains 3,200 mg. Omega-3 fatty acids, plus six grams of fiber of which 1,600 micrograms are cancer-fighting lignans. Flax seed oil has the perfect balance of Omega-6 and Omega-3 for our diet.

The National Cancer Institute is looking closely at flax for possible chemopreventive effects. Flax seeds are also one of nature's richest sources of lignans (also found in grains such as bran, buckwheat and corn). Lignans deactivate potent estrogens that can initiate the growth of cancerous tumors, especially in the breast and reproductive system. In fact, studies have shown that women who consume a diet high in lignans have lower rates of colon and breast cancer.

The best way to supplement flax is to grind up whole seeds (like in a grinder you would use for coffee beans) as you use them. After grinding, flax will only remain fresh for a day or so if kept in a small container in the refrigerator. You can add this to your salads, cottage cheese, yogurt, soups, cereals, etc. Be sure to add ground flax to cooked foods at the table, not the stove, as the high heat will destroy the integrity of the EFAs.

Using high-lignan flax seed oil is also an option.

Other nutrients provided by flax seeds include Vitamin E, beta carotene, calcium, magnesium, manganese and potassium. Flax seeds also contain high quality protein.

What to do with freshly ground flax seeds:

- Mix with non-fat yogurt, cottage cheese, cheese dips, etc. (the fiber helps the body rid itself of fat, especially saturated fats found in many dairy products).

- Mix into meat loaf, meat balls, soy balls, etc.

- Mix into homemade breads, waffles, muffins or other baked goods.

- Sprinkle onto salads, scrambled eggs, breakfast cereal (hot or cold), rice and steamed vegetables.

- Blend into fruit shakes with nonfat yogurt.

It is important to realize that the fatty acids in flax seeds are highly susceptible to destruction and rancidity by exposure to heat, light and oxygen. This is why it is important to buy whole flax seeds and grind them in a blender or coffee bean grinder and use them freshly ground.

Garlic and Onions

Garlic and onions have lipid-lowering and anti-clotting properties which protect us against heart disease and also contain sulfides that seem to protect against stomach cancer. They stimulate enzymes within cells which detoxify cancer-causing chemicals.

Numerous research groups have demonstrated garlic's ability to significantly decrease LDL cholesterol and triglyceride, inhibit platelet aggregation (help prevent blood clots), inhibit proliferative (plaque promoting) activity, enhance vascular permeability, and provide antioxidant protection. Garlic compounds also stimulate the formation of glutathione an amino acid that detoxifies foreign chemicals and is a powerful antioxidant.

Ginger

Ginger is a common flavoring agent which has been used for thousands of years to treat numerous conditions including stomach aches, diarrhea, nausea, cholera, hemorrhaging, arthritis and toothaches.

In the U.S., ginger has been used primarily as a digestive aid to help relieve excess gas and bloating; an aid in nausea, vomiting, morning sickness and motion sickness; a diaphoretic (to induce sweating) and an appetite stimulant.

Ginger has a beneficial effect on our regulatory prostaglandins and has been shown to inhibit platelet aggregation (clogging), even more so than garlic or onions. Ginger also benefits our inflammatory regulatory processes which helps conditions such as arthritis, bursitis, tendonitis, injuries and also allergies and asthma.

Mangos, Apricots
and other beta-carotene-rich fruits

Beta-carotene, which is just one of about 50 different carotenoids, is effective against singlet oxygen. It is a "weak" antioxidant compared to Vitamins E and C. Beta-carotene, found in fruits and brightly colored vegetables, is one of the few carotenoids which can convert to Vitamin A, a fat-soluble antioxidant. Vitamin A is ineffective against certain types of free radicals.

Vitamin A is one of the body's foremost antioxidant protectors and is the principal nutrient responsible for the health of our mucous membranes. Vitamin A supplementation stimulates mucous production and keeps membranes well lubricated and strong. It also strengthens the integrity of your bowel wall to help protect you from absorbing large protein molecules.

Studies show that foods containing beta carotene are more effective in protecting us against cancer than beta carotene is alone as a supplement. Just a reminder that God knew what he was doing when he made these delicious fruits.

Studies also show that taking large amounts of only one type of phytonutrient, such as beta-carotene, may impair absorption of other carotenes and important nutrients, so it is very important to get a **wide variety** of these important nutrients. Fruits and vegetables in their natural form contain many more carotenoids than just beta carotene, such as lutein and zeaxanthin, which are very important for your eyes.

Mushrooms

Mushrooms are very low in calories (one-half cup of raw pieces has just nine calories and one-half cup of cooked just 21). Mushrooms are very high in potassium, low in sodium and contain a fair amount of B Vitamins.

Asian mushrooms are quickly gaining popularity for their ability to fight cancer, inhibit blood clotting and stimulate immunity. Reishi mushrooms have anti-cancer and anti-histamine properties making them beneficial for individuals with allergies.

Shiitake mushrooms have been extensively researched. They contain an anti-viral polysaccharide which stimulates the immune system to produce interferon which fights off cancerous cells. (Takehara) Shiitake mushrooms are used as an anti-cancer treatment in Japan and may also help lower cholesterol.

Oats

Oats are awesome. I think one of the simplest and healthiest things you can do for your body is to eat a bowl of steel cut oats for breakfast at least five mornings a week. Steel cut oats is the least processed way to consume oats. Oat meal is more highly processed and instant oats are the worst because they also add sugar and other chemicals we do not need. Steel cut oats may take a little longer to cook, but you can cook up a batch and then simply reheat the leftovers the next day. I like to add a little amaranth (discussed on page 204). You can also increase the variety of your mornings by adding raisins, chopped apple, orange rind, cinnamon, cardamom or other things.

Oats (and also barley) are rich in the complex carbohydrate fiber known as beta glucan. Research shows this substance helps regulates blood sugar so it is excellent for those who are diabetic or hypoglycemic. (Wood, Wursch Tappy)

Beta glucan is also an excellent immune system stimulant. It increases levels of white blood cells and encourages them to work harder to clean up debris and pathogens in the body. There is also evidence showing its ability to help us fight cancer and tumors. (Hoffman, Ito, Ross)

There is also research showing beta glucan helps regulate our cholesterol levels. (Uusitupa, Braaten, Lia, Bobek, Behall, Lovegrove)

My grandfather, who lived until the wonderful age of 94, ate oatmeal for breakfast almost everyday. He also often ate soft boiled eggs (the healthiest way to eat eggs). I have no idea what his cholesterol level was because he never went to the doctor. He was never sick. When I was a kid, I used to think my grandpa was the strongest man on earth. He was wonderful. After he retired (he was a plumber at the Air Force Base) he would still get up at five in the morning and shovel snow (they lived in North Dakota where we are always shoveling) for all his neighbors.

My grandfather also loved sweets. After he died, I remember commenting that it was a wonder that he never became diabetic because of all the sweets he used to eat. Must have been all those oats!

Yams/Sweet Potatoes

Yams and sweet potatoes are so good for us that it is a shame that so many only enjoy them a few times a year during the holidays. These two similar tubers (edible root-like structures) are rich in plant sterols (fat-like compounds), which block estrogen promotion of breast cancer activity and help block the fat and cholesterol absorption.

Dioscorea yams are known to contain a high amount of a progesterone-like substance believed to help many women's problems such as PMS and menopause.

In areas where yams are consumed in large amounts, such as the Nigerian Yoruba tribe, there seems to be a correlation with the high birth rate of twins - double the rate of anywhere else. Researchers noted that wealthier Yoruba people who have given up a tribal yam-based diet for a Western diet have fewer twins. It is suspected that the hormone-like substances in the yam stimulate the ovaries to release more than one egg. These hormone-like substances deserve more research to determine their full potential.

Sweet potatoes contain a number of polyphenol compounds, such as chlorogenic acid, which work together to create a powerful antioxidant effect.

Sweet potatoes are rich in natural protease inhibitors that prevent the spread of cancer in animal studies and have become popular for their ability to kill disease-producing viruses such as HIV.

Sweet potatoes are full of fiber which also helps us fight off cancer, maintain good colon health, and helps us keep excess weight off. They are also very high in the antioxidant beta-carotene, and rich in potassium, magnesium and folic acid.

Spinach

Spinach is loaded with important antioxidants like beta-carotene, lutein and zeaxanthin (also found in tomatoes, kale, parsley, celery, leeks, pumpkin, yellow, green and red peppers and Swiss chard). These carotenoids are especially recognized for their ability to protect us against macular degeneration, cataracts and lung and breast cancer.

Spinach is also rich in minerals such as iron, potassium, calcium and magnesium.

A note on lettuce: In choosing a lettuce, in general, the darker the green, the higher nutritional value it has. Romaine lettuce and spinach, for example, contain a higher content of minerals and phytonutrients compared to butter or iceburg lettuce.

Spirulina

Spirulina is a blue-green algae renowned for its high usable protein content (65%), which also contains a high concentration of vitamins, minerals, essential fatty acids, chlorophyll and other special nutrients. It is especially rich in beta-carotene, and numerous other carotenes, Vitamin B-12 and the other B Complex Vitamins, iron, essential trace minerals and gamma linoleic acid (GLA).

As a protein source, it is more concentrated than any other natural food and contains all essential amino acids (fish and meat contain 15-25%, soybeans contain 35%, dried milk contains 35%, peanuts contain 35%, and eggs contain 12%). Spirulina also contains many valuable non-essential amino acids. The protein content is easily digested and assimilated in the body.

GLA, a polyunsaturated essential fatty acid, promotes cholesterol normalization (Becker) and is a precursor to prostaglandin compounds. These hormones stimulate energy production, and therefore are very important for fat metabolism. Prostaglandins also boost the effectiveness of insulin.

Alfalfa

This is one of the richest food sources of vitamins and minerals. The minerals are in a balanced form which promotes absorption. Alfalfa provides a rich supply of fiber, which encourages naturally softer stools.

Alfalfa also contains high amounts of chlorophyll, a natural detoxicant which helps remove toxins from the body. In addition, alfalfa contains saponins. These help prevent the absorption of dietary fat through the stomach and intestinal wall. This substance has been shown to actually remove cholesterol from the blood stream. Even better, it reduces dangerous LDL cholesterol and increases levels of beneficial HDL cholesterol.

Alfalfa sprouts can be found in the produce department at the grocery store and are an excellent addition to salads or sandwiches. Alfalfa is also available as a dietary supplement. The suggested daily intake is 2,000 mg. with meals.

A Few Other Supplements Worth Mentioning:

Omega-3 Fatty Acids

Eicosapentaenoic acid (EPA) and decosahexaenoic acid (DHA) are the Omega-3 unsaturated fatty acids found in fish oils and flax seed. EPA and DHA affect the synthesis of important anti-inflammatory chemicals in the body. They also help lower blood fat levels. Increased intake of EPA/DHA has been shown in numerous studies to lower blood triglyceride and cholesterol levels, while raising the level of high-density lipoprotein (HDL), the "good" cholesterol.

The intake of dietary EPA/DHA is enhanced by eating flax seeds, and cold water fish, such as salmon, herring, mackerel, or sardines that feed on certain plankton, or by taking additional oil supplements.

These lipid-lowering effects, along with some benefits in reducing platelet aggregation and clotting potential, make the use of EPA/DHA very important in the treatment or prevention of cardiovascular disease or in anyone with high blood fats or low HDL. The decreased blood viscosity and lower fat levels help reduce the risk of heart attacks.

The mild anti-inflammatory effects may also be helpful for arthritis and other inflammatory conditions. In rheumatoid arthritis, EPA/DHA supplementation has been shown to reduce joint stiffness and soreness and to improve flexibility.

In general, as a preventive for cardiovascular disease, it is recommended that we eat a serving of cold-water fish two or three times weekly. For high blood fats, low HDL, or those with increased risk of cardiovascular disease, supplement 2,000 mg. of EPA/DHA twice daily. Higher amounts may be needed for cholesterol lowering effects. Also, for supplying the valuable Omega-3 fatty acids, cold-pressed flaxseed oil is an excellent and less expensive source. Use it on pasta, grains (like oatmeal or rice), in salads, cottage cheese, etc. It has a mild nutty, buttery taste.

MSM

MSM (Methyl-sulfonyl-methane) is organic sulfur. Sulfur is the third (ties with potassium) largest existing mineral in the body, following calcium and phosphorus. This seems to surprise a lot of people as we don't seem to hear about the need for sulfur like we do many of the other minerals. We actually need much less zinc and chromium than we need sulfur.

While sulfur is present in every cell of the body, it is found in highest concentration in connective tissues such as cartilage, collagen and elastin. Sulfur bonds are an important structural component of all connective tissue. Connective tissue is found everywhere in the body – especially the joint tissues, mucus membranes – the lungs, sinus cavity, mouth, etc., and our skin. It supports and connects our internal organs, forms the walls of blood vessels, and joins muscles to bones. Collagen holds water and gives connective tissue its flexibility.

The body uses sulfur as a structural component (in combination with other nutrients, especially Vitamin C and amino acids) to continually create new healthy cells to replace old ones. If the body isn't receiving the proper nutrition for this process including sulfur, the body instead will produce weak dysfunctional cells. Scar tissue is an excellent visual example of the result of inadequate nutritional support as the body is trying to repair itself.

Sulfur is found in garlic, onions, cabbage, eggs, meat and some amino acids.

The following benefits have been demonstrated by MSM supplementation:

- Improves joint flexibility, reduces stiffness and swelling of arthritis-like conditions.

- Improves circulation and cell vitality.

- Reduces pain associated with systemic inflammatory disorders such as arthritis.

- Reduces scar tissue which further aggravates arthritis-like conditions, increasing pain and decreasing mobility.

- Breaks up calcium deposits: Arthritis may be induced by excess calcium as it can migrate to soft tissues and form deposits. The tissues become calcified and the cells cease to function normally. MSM is able to rupture the weak (water) bonds of calcium in the synovial fluid.

This is likely to also be true for kidney stones.

- Reduces allergies: MSM fortifies the body's natural barriers against allergens. Oral MSM has alleviated the allergic response to pollen and to foods. MSM is as good as or better than the traditional antihistaminic preparations, but without the side effects.

- Improves asthma: MSM also strengthens the lungs against allergic responses. It helps regulate the fluid covering the airway surface.

- Reduces snoring.

- Improves skin tone and reduce scars.

- Reduces nasal congestion (sinusitis).

- Improves digestive disorders, i.e., constipation, diverticulitis, ulcerative colitis, Crohn's disease, parasites, etc.

- Improves oral tissues (gum disease). (Zentner)

Golfers, joggers, tennis buffs, baseball players and athletes of all kinds all greatly appreciate the pain relief they get from MSM. It simply helps keep joints flowing smoothly.

Deficiency symptoms include slow wound healing, scar tissue and joint disorders such as arthritis and skin problems. In the last few years, MSM has become a highly popular nutritional supplement as it is so beneficial for so many people.

Colostrum

Colostrum, also known as "first milk," is the immune-enhancing fluid produced by all mammals at the time of birthing before milk is produced. This fluid is crucial to the survival and immune development of the newborn.

The immune factors in colostrum can also benefit adults. Colostrum from other animals such as cows, is highly beneficial for humans. While the mother cow produces 2.5-3 gallons of colostrum, the newborn can only consume about one-half gallon. If not consumed, the colostrum is reabsorbed by the mother.

For centuries many diary farmers utilized the excess colostrum in their family, making a custard-like dish out of it, providing an important immune boost in the early spring. These families boasted of having very few or no health problems. It seems that God does have a purpose for everything, but many of these important and valuable traditions have been lost with modernization.

Colostrum, rich in its immune-regulatory factors and other vital immune-supporting nutrients, is beneficial for many disorders such as allergies, colds and flu, arthritis, lupus, irritable bowel and other digestive problems. Colostrum also contains anti-inflammatory agents, which offer relief to individuals with arthritis.

Antioxidants

Antioxidants are nutrients which protect us from free radical damage. Researchers around the world tell us that free radical damage throughout the body is a major cause of aging and age-associated diseases.

A free radical is an incomplete, unstable molecule. It is incomplete because it is missing an electron, which exists in pairs in stable molecules. It is unstable because it will "steal" an electron from another molecule, and thereby create another free radical and a chain reaction of events, which results in thousands of reactions.

Every time molecules lose or gain an electron, they are weakened and, ultimately, the whole structure, whether it is an enzyme, protein, cell membrane, tissue or organ is damaged. Some areas of the body are more susceptible to damage than others. In their search for electrons, free radicals do a great deal of structural damage to healthy cells. Injured cells cannot function properly and may even die.

Production of oxygen free radicals is a normal part of the body's mechanism. They are produced as cells use oxygen to convert food into energy. There are tens of thousands of free radicals formed in the body every second. However, they are not all harmful; some actually help us. The body's immune system uses free radicals to kill potentially infectious microbes and viruses. This activity (called phagocytosis) however, at the same time, creates even more free radicals (hydrogen peroxide and hydroxyl radicals) that may lead to severe tissue damage.

Free radical damage is now widely known to shorten life. Free radicals are major factors in about 80 different diseases, including: (Ames)

Heart disease and stroke	Cancer (all types)
Diabetes	Cataracts
Macular degeneration	Allergies
Arthritis	Asthma
Lupus	Pancreatitis
Neuropathy	M.S.
Inflammatory bowel disease	Infections
Parkinson's disease	Gum disease
Other inflammatory conditions	

Alzheimer's and other neuro-degenerative diseases

In fact, researchers now agree that most common ailments, including virtually all chronic degenerative diseases, are caused either directly by or are closely associated with free radical damage.

Free Radicals Accelerate Aging. Aging also results from the loss of vital cells from free radical reactions. Prolonged exposure to free radicals fast-forwards the aging process. Free radicals turn the elastic, flexible tissues of youth into the wrinkled skin, stiff joints and hardened arteries of old age. In arterial cells, free radical damage reduces flexibility, which in turn raises blood pressure and puts extra strain on the heart as it pumps harder to maintain a continuous flow of blood. In the brain, free radicals impede message transmission between nerve cells, interfering with quick thinking, memory and concentration.

Free radicals' most damaging effects are upon the genetic material of our cells – DNA molecules. When these molecules are damaged, DNA replication is impaired. The entire process of renewal in the body depends on cells being able to replicate themselves exactly. Malformed cells may become cancerous if the immune system does not get rid of them.

Antioxidants are a class of nutrients that prevent the damage and diseases associated with free radicals. They also help alleviate the symptoms and side-effects of many of these conditions. (Yamakoshi, Packer)

Examples of antioxidants include:

Vitamins A, C and **E**

Carotenoids such as **beta-carotene, lutein, etc.**

Minerals such as **selenium** and **zinc**

Herbs such as **ginkgo biloba** and **milk thistle**

Extracts such as **lipoic acid** and **procyanidins**

Low levels of antioxidants increase free radical activity and increase our risk of health problems. Therefore, the use of antioxidant supplements to scavenge free radicals can potentially decrease the risks of cancer, cardiovascular disease, cataracts, macular degeneration, neuropathy and other circulatory problems and the many other degenerative conditions. (Barber)

As long as the ratio of oxidants to antioxidants remains in balance, the negative effects of the free radicals can be controlled. When the balance becomes upset by excessive exposure to internal or external factors or a combination of both, the antioxidants produced by the body simply cannot cope with the increased amount of free radicals.

In addition to the free radicals we produce as a natural part of our metabolic process, other factors that increase free radical exposure and your need for antioxidants include:

- Exercise
- Stress
- Exposure to toxins such as pollutants, smog, tobacco smoke, alcohol, drugs and pesticides
- Illness, infection, inflammation, and many health problems — diabetes, arthritis, asthma
- Elevated blood lipids (especially LDL)
- Elevated blood sugar
- Many stimulants and metabolic enhancers such as caffeine and diet pills
- Radiation (including UV light)

Alpha Lipoic Acid

Alpha lipoic acid has several unique properties. It is both fat and water soluble, meaning it can protect both the inside and outside of our cellular membranes. Lipoic acid also has regenerative properties for other antioxidants such as Vitamins C and E and glutathione. Instead of getting "used up" after donating an electron, lipoic acid can recycle these antioxidants by offering them an electron. (Packer)

Lipoic acid demonstrates powerful therapeutic properties for diabetes and is used throughout Europe to treat and prevent polyneuropathy, cataracts and macular degeneration. (Packer)

Lipoic acid is naturally found in foods such as potatoes, carrots and yams.

...and the leaves of the tree were for the healing of the nations.

Revelation 22:2

Ginkgo Biloba

The Ginkgo biloba tree has existed on earth longer than any other tree. The species has survived some 200 million years of geological upheaval, as well as a dramatically changing climate. Not even the atomic bomb on Hiroshima was destructive enough to prevent a Ginkgo tree, the only plant remaining in the area, from putting forth new shoots in the following spring. Today, that tree is a national monument and flourishes in what was virtually the center of the explosion.

As people grow older, blood flow in the brain decreases, which means less food and oxygen for brain cells. Reduced brain circulation can mean dizziness, memory loss, tinnitus (ringing in the ears), macular degeneration (the most common cause of blindness in the elderly) and even deafness (cochlear deafness). (Castleman)

Studies show that the components in Ginkgo help protect the sensitive brain cells from free radical molecules. (Eckmann) Ginkgo passes through the blood brain barrier and therefore provides neuro-protective functions as well as throughout the body. (Smith)

Research on Ginkgo biloba has identified its many beneficial properties. It is a powerful antioxidant which protects us from depressed antioxidant levels and stress. (White)

Ginkgo is also important for the inhibition of platelet aggregation factor (PAF). PAF is associated with platelet clotting, allergic reactions and acute inflammation. Too much PAF can also inhibit proper functioning of the cardiovascular system. (Braquet, Pietri, Maitra)

Numerous studies show that Ginkgo biloba extract helps us to maintain adequate antioxidant nutrition for our brain to function, such as remembering where you put your keys or glasses, what you were supposed to pick up at the grocery store or the directions to a place you haven't been in a few months. (Stoll, Grassel)

Studies confirm its beneficial effect on brain functions which commonly accompany advanced age.

Procyanidins

Oligomeric Procyanidins (OPCs or procyanidins) which come from grape seed or pine bark extracts are very powerful antioxidants. Studies show that these extracts are more potent in their antioxidant abilities than Vitamins C and E, yet they provide antioxidant protection for and help Vitamins C and E work better in the body.

A large body of scientific research clearly demonstrates the beneficial effect procyanidins have on a variety of health problems including heart disease, circulatory disorders, neuropathy and premature aging.

Procyanidins effectively protect us from free radical damage on a cellular level. They also help maintain optimal levels of other important antioxidants in the body such as Vitamins C and E and glutathione. (Virgili, Rimbach)

Procyanidins spare Vitamin C and other antioxidants by helping them work better and longer in the body. Research also shows that procyanidins are even more effective than Vitamin C in protecting LDL (the bad cholesterol) from oxidation, which is involved in the development of plaque in our arteries. (Laplaud)

Water

Water, in sufficient quantities, plays a major role in our health. Water is, in fact, the most important nutrient, because we cannot live more than three to four days without it.

Water accounts for over two-thirds of our total body weight. We lose water through perspiration, respiration, and the biggest loss is through the manufacture of urine (and also feces) to flush out bodily waste. All this water has to be replaced -- every single day.

Water improves digestion and makes you feel full.

Water is a natural diuretic. If you are not consuming enough water daily, the cells will hold onto it and may cause you to feel bloated when you are actually dehydrated. Try to drink eight large glasses of pure water daily.

Tips For Everyday Eating

- Before eating or drinking anything, ask yourself if by doing so, it brings glory to God. (Is it feeding your fleshly desires or providing sound nutrition for the needs of the body?)

- Eat three small balanced meals every day. Do not skip meals, especially breakfast. Eating breakfast increases your resting metabolic rate for all day. Many believe that breakfast should be the largest meal of the day.

- Do not overeat. Tighten your belt before meals. Also try putting meals on smaller plates.

- Before your meal, have a cup of clear soup and eat a salad (with low calorie dressing – try balsamic vinegar or lemon juice and flax seed oil).

- Eat more fiber. Fruits, vegetables, whole grains, seeds and beans add bulk to the diet and make you feel full. They are also nutrient-dense compared to processed foods, which also helps reduce cravings.

- Eliminate sugar and other highly processed foods (white bread, pastries, etc.). Cut down on simple carbohydrates and empty calorie foods like sweets and alcohol.

- Avoid all saturated fat. Avoid fried foods, fatty meats and skin from chicken and processed fats containing trans-fatty acids.

- Eat slowly. Chew your food thoroughly.

- Use lemon juice, herbs and spices to flavor food instead of butter, high calorie dressings and toppings.

- Avoid commercial diets, liquid diets, etc., which can cause nutrient deficiencies and do not teach good eating habits.

- Don't allow "dangerous" snack foods in the home or workplace. Binging usually occurs at home so make these foods unavailable.

- If you are craving an "unhealthy" food, purchase the smallest amount possible to eliminate the possibility of emptying a large container of it in one sitting or look for low-fat or low-calorie versions of the same food. For example, instead of ice cream, choose low-fat ice milk or frozen non-fat yogurt.

- If you need to snack, eat healthy fresh fruits or vegetables (cauliflower, broccoli, cucumbers, mushrooms, celery, apples, oranges, etc.).

- Avoid artificial sweeteners, for example, those found in diet drinks. Artificial sweeteners are many times sweeter than sugar so they cause a craving for sweets. In addition, artificial sweeteners fool the body into thinking it has ingested sugar. As a result, your body releases extra insulin that can lead to weight gain.

- Drink at least eight glasses of pure water every day.

- **Remember to give thanks.** We should always ask God to bless nutritious foods for our bodies to strengthen and nourish us. He can't bless non-nutritious "junk food." If you eat it you have to be prepared to suffer the consequences.

And ye shall serve the LORD your God, and He shall bless thy bread, and thy water; and I will take sickness away from the midst of thee. Exodus 23:25

For every creature of God is good, and nothing to be refused, if it be received with thanksgiving: For it is sanctified by the word of God and prayer. 1 Timothy 4:4-5

I think this refers to foods in their wholesome and natural form as God created them – not necessarily as man has adulterated healthy foods into non-nutritious non-food items to satisfy our flesh.

We need to pray before each and every meal to receive blessing upon our food before we partake of it. We cannot expect benefit from our food without that blessing, and we have no reason to expect that blessing if we do not pray for it. Thus, we must give glory to God as our benefactor, and acknowledge our dependence upon him and our obligations to Him.

And He took the seven loaves and the fishes, and gave thanks, and brake them, and gave to His disciples, and the disciples to the multitude. Matthew 15:36

Resist Conformity

Resist conformity to the world and embrace the transformation that comes in Jesus Christ. Many of you may be thinking:

"No one eats healthy like that."

"That healthy food would take too much work."

"I don't have time to prepare healthy meals."

"That kind of health food just doesn't taste good."

"Everyone eats at Mc--- or Burger----- or where ever."

...and probably dozens of other excuses. The Bible clearly tells us not to be conformed to this world. As Christians we are to be set apart from "what everyone else does."

And be not conformed to this world: but be ye transformed by the renewing of your mind, that ye may prove what is that good, and acceptable, and perfect, will of God. Romans 12:2

Be not conformed to this world warns us that the "world system" – the popular culture and manner of thinking (that is in rebellion against God) – will try to conform us to its ungodly pattern, and that process must be resisted. If the world thinks it is acceptable – in the eyes of God, it probably is not. Much of the world seems to feel that killing unborn children and that sex outside of marriage is acceptable too. If a non-nutritious diet high in sugar and fat, ladened with chemicals seems to be OK with the rest of world, why is this different?

The opposite of being *conformed to this world* is being *transformed by the renewing of your mind;* the battle ground between conforming to evil and a good transformation is within the mind of the believer. You can't live in the Spirit and the flesh at the same time. Christ said, *He that is not with me is against me; and he that gathereth not with me scattereth abroad* (Matthew 12:30).

So then because thou art lukewarm, and neither cold nor hot, I will spue thee out of my mouth. Revelation 3:16

Many people can look like they are "good Christians" on the outside, but actually have an inward life and manner of thinking that is offensive to God. God isn't satisfied with an external piety that can be seen only by men, but with who we really are on the inside.

Also, beware of the marketing gimmicks used to lure you and your children into eating at these places. Satan will use any means possible to rob you of your health!

A Note to Parents

I sometimes wonder if no one cooks any more. Picking up something at the drive-through does not replace a home-cooked meal. What kind of message are you giving to your children and family if you do not have the time to cook them a healthy, well-balanced meal? Mealtime is also an important time for family bonding. By allowing your children to eat "fast food" you are giving them a very loud message that it is OK to eat that way. It is very important to teach children how to eat and respect their bodies at a young age.

Train up a child in the way he should go: and when he is old, he will not depart from it. Proverbs 22:6

Sacrifice and Fasting

In the book of Daniel we see how he (Daniel) and the eunuchs piously refused to eat of the king's meat. They chose not to indulge their appetites with such dainties, to avoid the sinful, voluptuous pleasures of Babylon. They had learned David's prayer, *Let me not eat of their dainties* (Psalm 141:4), and Solomon's precept, *Be not desirous of dainties, for they are deceitful meat* (Proverbs 23:3), and accordingly formed their resolution. To excel in wisdom and piety, one must learn to keep body (and fleshly desires) under subjection.

Daniel suggested, *Prove us for ten days; during that time let us have nothing but pulse to eat, nothing but herbs and fruits, or parched peas or lentils, and nothing but water to drink, and see how we can live upon that, and proceed accordingly* (Daniel 1:13). People will not believe the benefits of a sparce diet, nor how much it contributes to the health of the body, unless they try it. A trial was accordingly conducted and Daniel and his fellows lived for ten days upon this sparce diet. At the end of the ten days they were compared with the other children, and were found *fairer and fatter in flesh, of a more healthful look and better complexion, than all those who did eat the portion of the king's meat.* They experienced wonderful improvement, above all their fellows, in health, wisdom and knowledge (Daniel 1:15-21).

If we do not give in to our fleshly desires, God does indeed have a special blessing for us. Keeping ourselves pure from the pollutions of sin is the way to have that comfort and satisfaction of health. The pleasures of sin are rottenness to the bones.

Daniel had a choice whether or not to eat the food everyone else was eating, and so do we. Many people would like to believe that the dietary principals outlined in the Old Testament are no longer valid because of the New Covenant we are under. It is true, we are no longer under the law, but the purpose of the law was for God's people to be Holy. *You shall be holy, for I the LORD your God am holy* (Leviticus 19:1).

Take a look at what the New Testament says about the Old Testament: *For whatsoever things were written aforetime were written for our learning, that we through patience and comfort of the scriptures might have hope* (Romans 15:4).

This holy character of God is the standard of life that the law holds forth for humanity. This is the standard written on our hearts and conscience (Romans 2:15).

I believe this includes feeding the body what is nutritious and helpful, and not toxic and detrimental. Base your food choices on these principals rather than on taste and fleshly desires. Stop eating when you are full. Learn to listen to the actual physical needs of your body rather than it's carnal indulgence. Your good health will bless you for it. In time you will grow to appreciate the wholesome taste of God's intended food in it's natural form and you will not crave sweets, unhealthy fats and other detrimental foods.

God Wants Us Whole!

Jesus has all that we need. The complete resources of the Godhead that we need for personal wholeness reside in Him. *"For in Him dwells all the fullness of the Godhead bodily; and you are complete in Him, which is the head of all principality and power"* (Colossians 2: 9-10). In Him, all wisdom and knowledge are contained: *"in whom are hidden all the treasures of wisdom and knowledge"* (Colossians 2:3). Jesus is the very life that we are called to live: *"Christ who is our life"* (Colossians 3:4).

Many times when Jesus was healing the sick, He would use the term *whole* instead of *healed*. The word whole implies that there was more than physical healing taking place. *And Jesus said unto him, Go thy way; thy faith hath made thee whole. And immediately he received his sight, and followed Jesus in the way* (Mark 10:52). *And He said unto him, Arise, go thy way: thy faith hath made thee whole* (Luke 17:19).

To be whole in Christ is His true desire for us. The Greek meaning for the word *whole* refers to being healthy of both body and soul. *Whole* and *health* seem to almost be interchangeable words. The Greek Old Testament (The Septuagint) speaks of health 42 times and views "wholeness" as a divine gift. In the New Testament, "whole" is used in the Gospels in reference to Jesus as a victor over sin and suffering. He restores health by his word. *Then saith He to the man, Stretch forth thine hand. And he stretched it forth; and it was restored whole, like as the other* (Matthew 12:13). *And He said unto her, Daughter, thy faith hath made thee whole; go in peace, and be whole of thy plague* (Mark 5:34).

By making the whole person healthy, Jesus creates new life that releases us not only from the burden of physical problems but the scars created by emotional suffering. This is truly what He wants for us.

To achieve this:

- **We must seek God and put Him first in our lives.**

- **We must have a personal relationship with Him.**

- **We must listen and be obedient to His word, His will, and the promptings of the Holy Spirit.**

This is a process. Although when some people come to know Christ as their savior, there are many dramatic and instant life changing events. After this, there is still a progression of molding and shaping for growth in Him. For others, such as myself, it is a slow, life-long process of growth.

A couple of weeks after I started writing this book,

I was listening to one of the individuals giving his testimony about the incredible healings in his life. I remember thinking, "I wish God would heal me like that." That night, I again asked that God would heal my lungs like I knew He could. I just hate having to rely upon drugs. God knows this – I have been complaining about it since 1979 when I started using them to treat my asthma.

Around that same time, I decided to only take one-half of my normal prescribed theophylline dosage (one 200 mg. tablet every 12 hours). I have been doing this little experiment from time to time for years, just to see if I can get away with it. By the next dosage (or before) my lungs will tighten to the extent that I end up returning to a full dose. I usually do not have to look at a clock to know if I have gone beyond 14 hours since taking a dose. My lungs always tell me.

For those who are unfamiliar with theophylline, here is the short version of it's "wonders."

Uses: This medication improves breathing by opening air passages in the lungs. It is used in the treatment of asthma, chronic bronchitis and emphysema.

How To Take: This medication is best when taken on an empty stomach one hour before or two hours after meals. If stomach upset occurs, it may be taken with food. This medication works best if a constant level is maintained in the body. Do this by taking doses at evenly spaced intervals.

Side Effects: Dizziness, headache, light-headedness, heartburn, stomach pain, loss of appetite, anxiety, irritability, restlessness, nervousness, sleeplessness and frequent urination. Inform your doctor if you experience chest pain, rapid or irregular heart beat, confusion, severe stomach pain or breathing difficulties while taking this medication.

Precautions: Avoid drinking large amounts of beverages containing caffeine (coffee, tea, colas) or eating large amounts of chocolate. Caffeine can increase the side effects of this medication. Smoking affects this medication. Be sure to tell your doctor if you smoke or use nicotine or if you stop smoking. Your dose may need to be adjusted. This medication should be used during pregnancy only if clearly needed. Because small amounts of this drug appear in breast milk, consult with your doctor before breast-feeding. Tell your doctor your complete medical history especially if you are taking medicine (beta-blockers) for high blood pressure. (Bender)

Theophylline is a cardiac stimulant similar to caffeine. This is the reason individuals using theophylline are advised not to consume additional caffeine. If you do, be ready for heart palpitations, headaches, hand tremors, shakiness and all of the other side effects listed earlier. Here is what one study reported:

"...marked adverse effects were encountered in the repeated dose phase (of theophylline administration), possibly related to unpleasant side-effects. Both EEG and EMG findings indicative of stimulation were associated with a single dose of theophylline, but substantial tolerance developed during four weeks of therapy.

These findings demonstrate CNS stimulation by both single and repeated doses of theophylline with the occurrence of adverse side-effects during repeated administrations. (Bartel)

I never wanted to take these drugs – I hate drugs. What are these drugs doing to my liver? How could I ever feel safe about having children if I was taking these drugs? Studies on both drugs report an increase in still-births, miscarriages and low-birthweight infants. (Gilbert) Both drugs are excreted in the breast milk. But, upon inquiry, the doctors always assured me that these were *"the safest drugs around – they have been around for decades."* I knew better. I had already done the research.

I learned years ago to check things out for myself where the medical field is concerned, not to believe everything told to me by doctors. Look things up for yourself on the internet, in a Physicians Desk Reference (PDR), Drug Facts book or other reference books.

The data on asthma deaths is quite alarming. Several reports indicate that asthma mortality has increased during the last few decades. It seems that the deaths may be actually not so much due to the asthma attack, but due to the adverse effects of the drugs used to try to stop the asthma attack. (Jorgensen, Robin, Hida)

"...three asthmatic children were dead on arrival at the local emergency room. All three had been treated with beta-2 agonist inhalation on a regular basis, without anti-inflammatory treatment,

Two of the children died while inhaling the beta-2 agonist." (Bibi)

In 1994 *Clinical Pharmacological Therapeutics* reported the dangerous effects of Isoproterenol, a beta-2 agonist similar to commonly prescribed albuterol inhalers such as Proventil®, Ventolin® and Serevent® (which is longer lasting and used more as a preventative). Beta-2 agonist drugs are bronchial dilators which open up the airways during an attack.

Beta-2 agonist drugs increase the heart rate and blood pressure, plus they have other effects that actually increase the need for oxygen by the body. During an attack, with constricted airways, the asthmatic is not able to inhale oxygen into the body. The combination can result in oxygen starvation (hypoxemia). *"Isoproterenol and hypoxemia-hypercapnia will increase myocardial oxygen demand and could prove to be detrimental in severe asthma."* (Bremner)

In experiencing an asthma attack, one becomes accustomed to using the inhaler for relief. If relief does not follow, one may keep using the inhaler in hopes that it will help bring the desperately needed oxygen into the body, without realizing it is actually making the situation worse.

Did anyone ever tell me not to keep using my inhaler during an attack if it was not working? NEVER. Do doctors EVER tell you that using your inhaler too much during a severe attack could kill you? Not likely – they seem to think they are the safest drugs around.

These inhalers are prescribed to children as young as four years old... and without warning to the parents.

Did you know that on average, the elderly take 14 prescription medications daily? This is insane. These drugs merely suppress symptoms, and few, with rare exceptions, deal with eliminating the underlying cause or causes of the difficulty. Many of these increase nutritional problems, which further aggravates health problems.

All this confirms what I always knew. There *has* to be a better way.

Getting back to my story... Without giving it much thought, I continued to take one-half dosages for the next day or so. A few days passed and I realized I had not been using my inhaler so decided to stop taking the drug altogether. Later that day it finally dawned on me that God had given me new lungs! I have been taking that drug for over 20 years and have never been able to go longer than about 14 hours without my lungs tightening. I HAVE NEW LUNGS! I am completely free of all medications.

You just never know what God is going to do. When you pray, you have to expect miracles, because miracles do happen when you put God in charge of your whole life.

Is it a coincidence that the circumstances of the last several years of my life had been such that there was nothing I could do but cry out to Him? Absolutely not! That was what He wanted me to do all along. When life is going along fine, too many of us get so caught up in our lives that we lose focus of what is really important: Him. He just may allow our circumstances to get so bad that we have no choice but to go back to Him, where we belong. That's why He healed me. I finally went home.

He wants us all home. If we are lost, He will search for us and bring us back one by one doing whatever it will require for us to seek Him. That's how much He loves us. God wants us well.

> ***Their soul shall be as a watered garden;***
> ***and they shall not sorrow any more at all.***
> **Jeremiah 31:12**

The Last Chapter: Becoming Whole

Wholeness involves not only physical healing, but requires the healing of the soul. The soul is our connection with the world and with man. It involves our emotions – love, happiness, hurt, pain, suffering, anger, fear, anxiousness, etc. A soul tie is created with people we are close to and have relationships with – parents and family, friends, spouse, children, etc.

A negative (ungodly) soul tie is created when these relationships become abusive and involve sin. This can include any kind of physical, sexual or psychological abuse resulting in the pain and suffering of our soul. Unless these ungodly soul ties are severed or healed, the door for Satan to use these ties against you is open. He will "pull on the ties of those connections" continuing to make you feel guilty, angry, fearful, anxious, insecure, inadequate, or miserable and suffering as long as you let him. As long as you let the world beat you up, Satan has a hold on you. _This interferes with your relationship with God_. You must _let go_ of the pain and suffering from the past in order to maintain or obtain a proper relationship with God. When you do this, you can be whole; you can be well.

Christ died on the cross for us and experienced all the pain and suffering that we have ever experienced in our whole life all at once. Unless we let go of our pains, it is like we are telling Him that what He did was for nothing. Our sins are already paid for; you do not have to continue to beat yourself up.

We can be physically well, but still have pain in our souls. Or, we may still suffer from the pain of arthritis, cancer, heart disease, asthma, or any other ailment, and be free in our soul. If we can be free in our soul, our spirit (our connection to God), can be free and we can be healed. Our relationship with God is what is most important.

There is a scripture that has always concerned me.

Not every one that saith unto me, Lord, Lord, shall enter into the kingdom of heaven; but he that doeth the will of my Father which is in heaven. Many will say to me in that day, Lord, Lord, have we not prophesied in Thy name? and in Thy name have cast out devils? and in Thy name done many wonderful works? And then will I profess unto them, I never knew you: depart from me, ye that work iniquity. Matthew 7:21-23

This tells me there are people (believers) who think they are "saved" – going to heaven, but are not. In trying to understand what is meant by *"not everyone shall enter into the kingdom of heaven,"* I realized there are two important parts to this passage.

1. We must do the will of God, *"but he that <u>doeth the will of my Father</u> which is in heaven."*

2. We must have a personal relationship with God, *"I never <u>knew</u> you."*

If we do not have an intimate and personal relationship with God, there is no way for us to know what God's will is for us. A personal relationship with anyone (including God) takes time, develops over time and requires that the two involved (you and God) spend time together. Just as if you want to have a good relationship with your children, you have to spend time together. It is not enough to live under the same roof together, you must spend time talking with each other and doing things together. It is the same with God.

If you are a new Christian and have only recently accepted Christ as your personal savior, or even if you have been a Christian a long time, but do not have a personal relationship with God, you may wonder how to know what God's will is for you and how to have a personal relationship with God.

Husbands, love your wives, even as Christ also loved the church (body of believers)*, and gave himself for it; That he might sanctify and cleanse it with the washing of water **by the word**.* Ephesians 5:25-26

The best way to get to know God is to spend time

in His Word. We are to read it. We are to meditate on it. We are to hide His words in our heart. We are able to know the true and living God through His Word as it reveals God's character and His plan for mankind. It is through reading His Word that we come to a knowledge of the righteousness of God and that which He requires of us.

It is also the best place to go if we are hurting. Only God knows exactly how you feel and how much you are suffering. He is the only one who has been there with you experiencing all that you have gone through in your whole life – every step of the way.

You can talk to counselors and other people (even other Christians) till you are blue in the face, but you will never find anyone to completely understand your hurts and needs. You will be judged, you will be misunderstood. You have to go to God.

My soul melteth for heaviness: strengthen thou me according unto thy word. Psalms 119:28

This is my comfort in my affliction: for thy word hath quickened me. Psalms 119:50

When you are hurting, the Psalms are a great place to go. Not just because David, the author of many of the Psalms, was a sinner like us, but because David also knew God. God claimed David was a man after his own heart. Psalm 119 is an excellent devotional on the word of God.

If you don't understand the scriptures, just keep reading. If you truly want to understand it and pray that the Holy Spirit reveal the meaning to you, He will. Be patient. It took me a long time (and I still have a lot to learn). I know He will do the same for you. It is a process – it does not happen overnight.

I accepted Christ as my personal savior when I was 17 years old, but after that spent many years running around lost. I was still trying to live in the world – and had to suffer the consequences of everything that went along with it. I may have even been searching... going to church, Bible study, reading, etc., but until that time comes, when we start truly living in the Spirit, we are missing out on the true blessings of God.

Verily, verily, I say unto thee, Except a man be born of water and of the Spirit, he cannot enter into the kingdom of God... The wind bloweth where it listeth, and thou hearest the sound thereof, but canst not tell whence it cometh, and whither it goeth: so is every one that is born of the Spirit (John 3:5,8).

We must strengthen our spirit with the Word of God. The stronger the spirit, the more we are able to understand what God wants of us (to live in the spirit) verses doing what we what (to live in the flesh). A damaged, hurting soul will interfere with your spirit and your relationship to God.

God may heal you physically in an instant, but sometimes the healing of the soul takes longer – and may be much more painful and difficult. Sometimes these hurts and pains (from rejection, abuse, domestic violence, divorce, death of a parent, spouse or child, parental abandonment, rape, incest, dysfunctional homes and relationships formed due to alcoholism or other forms of addiction, etc.) are carried with us for a lifetime. We will hold onto them and continue to beat ourselves up until we finally realize that the price **has been paid!**

You are loved, you are worthy, you are just as important to God as the next person. Christ died for all of us.

But He was wounded for our transgressions, He was bruised for our iniquities: the chastisement of our peace was upon Him; and with his stripes we are healed. Isaiah 53:5

Confess your faults one to another, and pray one for another, that ye may be healed. The effectual fervent prayer of a righteous man availeth much. James 5:16

If you have confessed your sin and asked God for forgiveness, have **repented** from your ways, and have forgiven the individuals (all of them) who have hurt you, then there is nothing else to do. Let go!

And it shall come to pass in that day, that his burden shall be taken away from off thy shoulder, and his yoke from off thy neck, and the yoke shall be destroyed because of the anointing. Isaiah 10:27

Jesus said: *The Spirit of the Lord is upon me, because He hath anointed me to preach the gospel to the poor; He hath sent me to heal the broken-hearted, to preach deliverance to the captives, and recovering of sight to the blind, to set at liberty them that are bruised.* Luke 4:18

God wants you well. I want you well. I know how hard it is to not feel well and to be totally beat up by the world. I want you to experience the same freedom in Christ that I now have. I want to pray for you:

Father, in the name of our savior Christ Jesus, I ask for a complete healing of this individual. It is written that a prayer of faith will save the sick and the Lord will raise him up. I ask forgiveness of all sins that may have been committed and ask that you would be faithful in calling to attention any unconfessed sin that needs to be addressed.

Lord, you were pierced for our sin, you bore all our pain and suffering on that cross. We know that only through you and because of what you have done may we be completely healed and whole.

I thank you for this person and the miracle that you have created in them and the work that they are doing for you. I ask that you continue to draw this person to you, to strengthen them and to give them the peace and joy that only can be obtained through you. I thank you for this new day of freedom through you.

He Himself bore our sins in His body on the tree, so that we might die to sins and live to righteousness: by His wounds you have been healed. 1 Peter 2:24

Bibliography

Ames BN; Shigenaga MK; Hagen TM Oxidants, antioxidants, and the degenerative diseases of aging. Division of Biochemistry and Molecular Biology, University of California, Berkeley 94720. Proc Natl Acad Sci U S A 1993 Sep 1;90(17):7915-22

Barber, D.A., Harris, S.R., Oxygen free radicals and antioxidants: a review. Department of Surgery, Mayo Clinic & Foundation, Rochester, Minn.Am Pharm 1994 Sep;NS34(9):26-35.

Bartel P; Delport R; Lotz B; Ubbink J; Becker P; Effects of single and repeated doses of theophylline on aspects of performance, electrophysiology and subjective assessments in healthy human subjects. Neuropsychopharmacology Laboratory, HF Verwoerd Hospital Pretoria, South Africa. Psychopharmacology (Berl) 1992;106(1):90-6.

Behall KM, Scholfield DJ, Hallfrisch J; Effect of beta glucan level in oat fiber extracts on blood lipids in men and women. J Am Coll Nutr 1997;16(1)46-51.

Bender B; Milgrom H. Theophylline-induced behavior change in children. An objective evaluation of parents' perceptions. Department of Pediatrics, National Jewish Center for Immunology and Respiratory Medicine, Denver, CO 80206. JAMA 1992 May 20;267(19):2621-4.

Bibi H; Mahamid J; Shoseyov D; Armoni M; Liss Z; Schlesinger M; [Sudden death from asthma in childhood, is it preventable?] Pediatrics Dept., Barzilai Medical Center, Ashkelon. Harefuah 1998 Apr 15;134(8):609-10, 671.

Block, Gladys, et al "Fruit, Vegetable and Cancer Protection: A Review of the Epidemiological Evidence," Nutrition and Cancer, 1992, Vol 17: 2, 1-29.

Bobek P; Galbavy S; The oyster mushroom (Pleurotus ostreatus) effectively prevents the development of atherosclerosis in rabbits] Vyskumny ustav vyzivy, Bratislava. Ceska Slov Farm 1999 Sep;48(5):226-30

Bobek P; Galbavy S; Hypocholesterolemic and antiatherogenic effect of oyster mushroom (Pleurotus ostreatus) in rabbits. Research Institute of Nutrition, Bratislava, Slovak Republic.Nahrung 1999 Oct;43(5):339-42

Bobek P; Ozdin O; Mikus M; Dietary oyster mushroom (Pleurotus ostreatus) accelerates plasma cholesterol turnover in hypercholesterolaemic rat. Physiol Res 1995;44(5):287-91.

Braaten JT; Scott FW; Wood PJ; et al; High beta-glucan oat bran and oat gum reduce postprandial blood glucose and insulin in subjects with and without type 2 diabetes. Diabet Med 1994 Apr;11(3):312-8.

Braaten JT; Wood PJ; Scott FW; Wolynetz MS; etal; Oat beta-glucan reduces blood cholesterol concentration in hypercholesterolemic subjects. Eur J Clin Nutr 1994 Jul;48(7):465-74.

Brawley OW; Parnes H; Prostate cancer prevention trials in the USA. National Cancer Institute, 6120 Executive Boulevard, EPS 320, Bethesda, MD. Eur J Cancer 2000 Jun;36(10):1312.

Bremner P; Burgess C; McHaffie D; Robinson B; Galletly D; Buckly D; Beasley R; Purdie G; Crane J. The effect of hypercapnia and hypoxemia on the cardiovascular responses to isoproterenol. Department of Medicine, Wellington School of Medicine, New Zealand. Clin Pharmacol Ther 1994 Sep;56(3):302-8.

Estrada A; Yun CH; Van Kessel A; et al. Immunomodulatory activities of oat beta-glucan in vitro and in vivo. Microbiol Immunol 1997;41(12):991-8

Christen, W.G,. Manson, J.E., Seddon, J.M,. Glynn, R.J,. Buring, J.E., Rosner, B., Hennekens, C.H., A prospective study of cigarette smoking and risk of cataract in men. Channing Laboratory, Department of Medicine, Harvard Medical School, Boston, MA. JAMA 1992 Aug 26;268(8):989-93.

Diplock AT Antioxidant nutrients and disease prevention: an overview. Am J Clin Nutr 1991 Jan;53(1 Suppl):189S-193S

Erasmus, Udo. Fats and Oils (1986) Alive Books, Vancouver, British Columbia, Canada.

Franceschi S; Favero A; The role of energy and fat in cancers of the breast and colon-rectum in a southern European population. Servizio di Epidemiologia, Centro di Riferimento Oncologico, Aviano, Italy. Ann Oncol 1999;10 Suppl 6:61-3.

Gilbert SG; Rice DC; Reuhl KR; Stavric B, Adverse pregnancy outcome in the monkey (Macaca fascicularis) after chronic caffeine exposure. Toxicology Research Division, Health and Welfare Canada, Tunney's Pasture, Ottawa, Ontario. J Pharmacol Exp Ther 1988 Jun;245(3):1048-53.

Grassel E Effect of Ginkgo-biloba extract on mental performance. Double-blind study *using computerized measurement conditions in patients with cerebral insufficiency* Fortschr Med 1992 Feb 20;110(5):73-6

Guthrie N; Carroll KK; Specific versus non-specific effects of dietary fat on carcinogenesis. Department of Biochemistry, University of Western Ontario, London, Canada. Prog Lipid Res 1999 May;38(3):261-71.

Henry, M.; Matthew Henry's Consise Commentary on The Whole BobleThomas Nelson Publishers, Nachville, TN, 1997.

Hida W, Role of ventilatory drive in asthma and chronic obstructive pulmonary disease. First Department of Internal Medicine, Tohoku University School of Medicine, Sendai, Japan. Curr Opin Pulm Med 1999 Nov;5(6):339-43.

Hocman G Prevention of cancer: vegetables and plants. Research Institute of Preventive Medicine, Bratislava, Czechoslovakia. Comp Biochem Physiol [B] 1989; 93(2):201-12

Hoekstra, B; "The God of All Grace Developing Our Lives" Day By Day By Grace Daily Devotional, Blue Letter Bible. Nov. 26th 2000.

Hoffman OA, Olson EJ, Limper AH Fungal beta-glucans modulate macrophage release of tumor necrosis factor-alpha in response to bacterial lipopolysaccharide. Immunol Lett. 1993 Jul;37(1):19-25.

Hu FB; Rimm EB; Stampfer MJ; Prospective study of major dietary patterns and risk of coronary heart disease in men. Am J Clin Nutr 2000 Oct;72(4):912-21.

Hughes JA, West NX, Parker DM, van den Braak MH, Addy M; Effects of pH and concentration of citric, malic and lactic acids on enamel, in vitro. J Dent 2000 Feb;28(2):147-52.

Hughes JR; McHugh P; Holtzman S; Caffeine and schizophrenia.   Psychiatr Serv 1998 Nov;49(11):1415-7

Ito H, Shimura K, Itoh H, Kawade M; Antitumor effects of a new polysaccharide-protein complex (ATOM) prepared from Agaricus blazei (Iwade strain 101) "Himematsutake" and its mechanisms in tumor-bearing mice. Anticancer Res 1997 Jan-Feb;17(1A):277-84.

Jorgensen IM; Bulow S; Jensen VB; Dahm TL; Prahl P; Juel K; Asthma mortality in Danish children and young adults, 1973-1994: epidemiology and validity of death certificates. Dept of Paediatrics, Gentofte University Hospital, Copenhagen, Denmark. Eur Respir J 2000 May;15(5):844-8.

Kaul L; Nidiry J "High-fiber diet in the treatment of obesity and hypercholesterolemia" J Natl Med Assoc 1993 Mar;85(3):231-2.

Kimball, SR., Jefferson IS, Diabetes Metab Rev 4:773 (1988)

Lia A; Hallmans G; Sandberg AS; Sundberg B; et al; Oat beta-glucan increases bile acid excretion and a fiber-rich barley fraction increases cholesterol excretion in ileostomy subjects.Am J Clin Nutr 1995 Dec;62(6):1245-51

Liu S; Manson JE; Lee IM; Cole SR; Hennekens CH; Willett WC; Buring JEFruit and vegetable intake and risk of cardiovascular disease: the Women's Health Study. Division of Preventive Medicine and Channing Laboratory, the Department of Medicine, Brigham and Women's Hospital and Harvard Medical School, Boston, MA Am J Clin Nutr 2000. Oct;72(4):922-8

Lovegrove JA; Clohessy A; Milon H; Williams CM; Modest doses of beta-glucan do not reduce concentrations of potentially atherogenic lipoproteins. Am J Clin Nutr 2000 Jul;72(1):49-55.

Mensink, Ronald P. and Martijn B. Katan, "Effect of Dietary Trans-fatty Acids on High Density and Low Density Lipoprotein Cholesterol Levels in Healthy Subjects," New England Journal of Medicine (16 Aug 1990) 323 (7): 439-445.

Nayaka, N. el al, "Cholesterol lowing effect of spirulina" Tokai University, Japan. Nutrition Reports Int'l, June 1988, Vol 37:6 132901337.

Nelson GJ; Schmidt PC; Bartolini GL; Kelley DS; Kyle D; The effect of dietary docosahexaenoic acid on plasma lipoproteins and tissue fatty acid composition in humans. USDA, San Francisco, California Lipids 1997 Nov;32(11):1137-46.

Netzer, Corinne, The Complete Book Of Food Counts, Dell Publishing, NY, New York (1991).

Ornquist, Bryan, Lakes Area Vineyard Church, email dated 1/06/01, Detroit Lakes, MN

Packer L., Suzuki, "Vitamin E and Alpha-Lipoate: Role in Antioxidant Recycling and Activation of the NF-KB Transcription Factor" Molec. Aspects med. (1993).

Pietri S; Maurelli E; Drieu K; Culcasi M Cardioprotective and anti-oxidant effects of the terpenoid constituents of Ginkgo biloba extract (EGb 761). J Mol Cell Cardiol 1997 Feb;29(2):733-42

Maitra I; Marcocci L; Droy-Lefaix MT; Packer L Peroxyl radical scavenging activity of

Ginkgo biloba extract EGb 761. Biochem Pharmacol 1995 May 26;49(11):1649-55.

Mazariegos-Ramos E; Guerrero-Romero F; Rodriguez-Moran M; Lazcano-Burciaga G; Paniagua R; Amato D; Consumption of soft drinks with phosphoric acid as a risk factor for the development of hypocalcemia in children: a case-control study. J Pediatr 1995 Jun;126(6):940-2.

Rai GS; Shovlin C; Wesnes KA A double-blind, placebo controlled study of Ginkgo biloba extract ('tanakan') in elderly outpatients with mild to moderate memory impairment. Curr Med Res Opin 1991;12(6):350-5.

Rao, H. et al "Influence of beta-carotene on Immune Function" Carotenoids in Human Health, Ann NY Acad Sci, 1993, Vol 691, 262-264.

Robin ED, McCauley R. Sudden cardiac death in bronchial asthma, and inhaled beta-adrenergic agonists. Chest. 1992 Jun;101(6):1699-702.

Ross GD; Vetvicka V; Yan J; Xia Y; Vetvickova J Therapeutic intervention with complement and beta-glucan in cancer. Immunopharmacology 1999 May;42(1-3):61-74.

Siegel, B.; Peace, Love & Healing, Harper & Row Publishing, New York, 1989, pg. 179.

Smith W; Mitchell P; Leeder SR; Dietary fat and fish intake and age-related maculopathy. National Centre for Epidemiology and Population Health, Australian National University, Australian Capital Territory. Arch Ophthalmol 2000 Mar;118(3):401-4.

Stoll S; Scheuer K; Pohl O; Muller WE *Ginkgo biloba extract (EGb 761) independently improves changes in passive avoidance learning and brain membrane fluidity in the aging mouse.* Pharmacopsychiatry 1996 Jul;29(4):144-9.

Stoner GD; Mukhtar H Polyphenols as cancer chemopreventive agents. J Cell Biochem Suppl 1995;22:169-80.

Tappy L; Gugolz E; Wursch P; Effects of breakfast cereals containing various amounts of beta-glucan fibers on plasma glucose and insulin responses in NIDDM subjects. Diabetes Care 1996 Aug;19(8):831-4.

Tsuda H; et al., Chemopreventive effects of beta-carotene, alpha-tocopherol and five naturally occurring antioxidants on initiation of hepatocarcinogenesis by 2-amino-3-methylimidazo[4,5-f]quinoline. Jpn J Cancer Res 1994 Dec;85(12):1214-9.

Uusitupa MI; Miettinen TA; Sarkkinen ES; et al; Lathosterol and other non-cholesterol sterols during treatment of hypercholesterolaemia with beta-glucan-rich oat bran. Eur J Clin Nutr 1997 Sep;51(9):607-11.

Valenzuela A; Morgado N; Trans fatty acid isomers in human health and in the food industry. Laboratorio de Lipidos y Antioxidantes, INTA, Universidad de Chile, Santiago, Chile. Biol Res 1999;32(4):273-87.

Virgili F; Kim D; Packer L; Procyanidins extracted from pine bark protect alpha-tocopherol in ECV 304 endothelial cells challenged by activated RAW 264.7 macrophages: role of nitric oxide and peroxynitrite. University of California, Berkeley FEBS Lett 1998 Jul 24;431(3):315-8.

Virgili F; Kobuchi H; Packer L: Procyanidins extracted from Pinus maritima (Pycnogenol): scavengers of free radical species and modulators of nitrogen monoxide metabolism in activated murine RAW 264.7 macrophages, Free Radic Biol Med 1998 May;24(7-8):1120-9.

Walford RL; Harris SB; Gunion MW "The calorically restricted low-fat nutrient-dense diet in Biosphere 2 significantly lowers blood glucose, total leukocyte count, cholesterol, and blood pressure in humans." *Proc Natl Acad Sci U S A* 1992 Dec 1;89(23):11533-7.

Weisburger JH; Eat to live, not live to eat. Nutrition. 2000 Sep;16(9):767-73.

Wood PJ; Beer MU; Butler G; Evaluation of role of concentration and molecular weight of oat beta-glucan in determining effect of viscosity on plasma glucose and insulin following an oral glucose load. Br J Nutr 2000 Jul;84(1):19-23.

Wursch P; Pi-Sunyer FX; The role of viscous soluble fiber in the metabolic control of diabetes. A review with special emphasis on cereals rich in beta-glucan. Nestle Research Centre, Lausanne, Switzerland. Diabetes Care 1997 Nov;20(11):1774-80.

Wyshak G; Teenaged girls, carbonated beverage consumption, and bone fractures. Department of Psychiatry, Harvard Medical School, Boston, Arch Pediatr Adolesc Med 2000 Jun;154(6):610-3.

Yamakoshi J; Kataoka S; Koga T; Ariga T.; Proanthocyanidin-rich extract from grape seeds attenuates the development of aortic atherosclerosis in cholesterol-fed rabbits Atherosclerosis 1999 Jan;142(1):139-49.

Zentner A; Heaney TG An in vitro investigation of the role of high molecular weight human salivary sulphated glycoprotein in periodontal wound healing. J Periodontol 1995 Nov;66(11):944-55

ABOUT THE AUTHOR

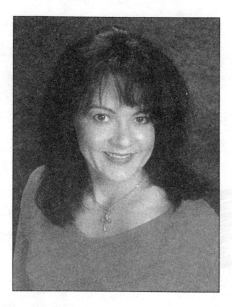

Beth M. Ley, Ph.D., has been a science writer specializing in health and nutrition for over 12 years and has written many health related books, including the best sellers, ***DHEA: Unlocking the Secrets to the Fountain of Youth*** and ***MSM: On Our Way Back to Health With Sulfur.*** She wrote her own undergraduate degree program and graduated in Scientific and Technical Writing from North Dakota State University in 1987 (combination of Zoology and Journalism). Beth has her masters (1997) and doctoral degrees (1999) in Nutrition.

Beth lives in the Minnesota lakes country. She is dedicated to God and to spreading the health message. She enjoys spending time with her dalmatian, exercises on a regular basis, eats a vegetarian, low-fat diet and takes anti-aging supplements.

Memberships: American Nutraceutical Association, American Academy of Anti-aging, New York Academy of Sciences, Oxygen Society.

ORDER THESE GREAT BOOKS
FROM BL PUBLICATIONS!

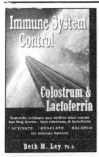

Immune System Control Colostrum & Lactoferrin
Beth M. Ley, Ph.D.
200 pages, $12.95

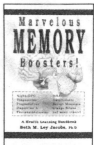

Marvelous Memory Boosters Beth M. Ley, Ph.D.
32 pages, $3.95

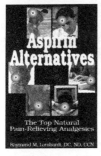

Aspirin Alternatives: The Top Natural Pain-Relieving Analgesics
Raymond Lombardi, D.C., N.D., C.C.N.,
160 pages, $8.95

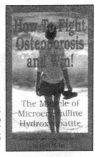

How to Fight Osteoporosis & Win: The Miracle of MCHC
Beth M. Ley, 80 pgs. $6.95

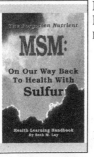

MSM: On Our Way Back To Health With Sulfur
Beth M. Ley, 40 pages, $3.95

Fading: One family's journey with a woman silenced by Alzheimer's w/ Preventative, Nutritional & Psychological Help for the Families & Patients with Alzheimer's
Frances Kraft, Dr. Barry Kraft, Dr. Beth Ley,
200 pgs. $12.95

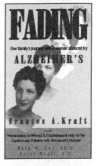

An excellent inspirational & resource book.

Bilberry & Lutein: The Vision Enhancers
Beth M. Ley, Ph.D. 40 pgs. $4.95

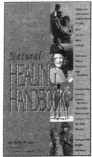

Natural Healing Handbook
Beth Ley 320 pgs. $14.95

TO PLACE AN ORDER:

Subtotal $ _____ Please add $4.00 for shipping. **TOTAL $** _____

Send check or money order to:

BL Publications 14325 Barnes Drive Detroit Lakes, MN 56501

Credit card orders call toll free: 1-877-BOOKS11

Also visit: www.blpbooks.com